IMAGES of America

NORTHAMPTON STATE HOSPITAL

On the Cover: This 1909 photograph of Northampton State Hospital (NSH) was taken from a specially erected tower, providing a unique angle on the hospital at its most physically impressive. (Courtesy of Historic Northampton.)

IMAGES
of America

NORTHAMPTON STATE HOSPITAL

J. Michael Moore and Anna Schuleit Haber

ARCADIA
PUBLISHING

ISBN 978-1-4671-2226-9

Published by Arcadia Publishing
Charleston, South Carolina

Printed in the United States of America

Library of Congress Control Number: 2014933350

For all general information, please contact Arcadia Publishing:
Telephone 843-853-2070
Fax 843-853-0044
E-mail sales@arcadiapublishing.com
For customer service and orders:
Toll-Free 1-888-313-2665

Visit us on the Internet at www.arcadiapublishing.com

For Mary, John, Kermit, Paul, and Bob

Contents

Acknowledgments 6

Introduction 7

1. Creation 9
2. Inertia 31
3. Change 79
4. Remembrance 113

ACKNOWLEDGMENTS

This book would not have been possible without the wonderful cooperation of Historic Northampton, including Kerry Buckley and Nan Wolverton, who generously provided access to its collections, and Marie Panik, who patiently answered many questions and provided gracious support over many visits. All of the images in this book, except where noted, are courtesy of Historic Northampton. We wish we were able to acknowledge all of the people who, over the decades, snapped, preserved, donated, and explained those photographs, but many of the photographers will never be known. Our special thanks go to Helen Sullivan, Betty Provost, Priscilla Hill, Myrtle Kuczenski, Mary Pelis, and Jackie Duda for their many insights in this regard.

Our understanding of the history of Northampton State Hospital has been enriched by the personal accounts of many people with an intimate connection to it. Some of these stories were collected in the year leading to the closing of the hospital in 1993, in a project that was advised by employees and funded by the Massachusetts Department of Mental Health. We would like to thank the many people who contributed to that effort. George Button Jr. worked especially hard to bring that project about and to make it a success. Stan Sherer is a gifted photographer, whose images have documented life in many contexts, including Northampton State Hospital in the year that it closed. We thank him for donating the use of several of his eloquent images of the hospital and its people. Michael Moore would like to thank David Glassberg for getting him in the door of the hospital and for his many kindnesses since.

The history of mental health care in America is layered and multifaceted, and the writings of several scholars provided an invaluable guide to us in the writing of our text, including Gerald N. Grob, Phil Brown, David Rothman, John Maurice Grimes, and Albert Deutsch. Anyone seeking to understand this history will appreciate the debt we owe them.

We would also like to acknowledge those who further broadened our understanding of this specific hospital through their work, including Steven J. Schwartz and the Center for Public Representation, Michael Tillyer and the Anchor House of Artists, Cheryl Stevens, Rebecca Macauley, Steve Holochuck, Kerry Holland, James Duffy, Ken Duckworth, and Mary Pelis.

Our special thanks go to our families for their enduring support along this journey during the many hours we spent peering into the past and piecing fragments together into an incomplete narrative. Thank you all.

Introduction

Northampton State Hospital was a public facility, established and paid for by the citizens of Massachusetts to care for, treat, and cure people with serious mental illness. This was a revolutionary idea when the hospital was established in 1856. Even today, the complex range of conditions called mental illness is little understood. But in a typically American attitude that combined a conviction of the efficacy of human action with a utopian vision of the perfectibility of society, the task was undertaken.

In the United States, the discipline of psychiatry was created by a group of men who built and ran asylums. The foundation of these asylums was order, the order that would heal a disordered mind. Regularity, routine, and punctuality were built into the very physical structures, structures that were standardized in the decade before the hospital in Northampton was built. The hospital here, like more than 50 others across the country, was designed to this standard. But prisons are built on order, and order was not enough to effect a cure. Beauty was the inspiration for a happy life, and beautiful settings and grounds would project the harmony of nature to the spirit of the inmates. Once the "demons" of mental illness had been harnessed, a person could respond to the natural call for human fellowship and society. So the asylum would have ample means for the exercise of body and mind. There were farms and gardens to work and lectures and religious services to attend. Rational minds, healthy bodies, and serene spirits would be the prize.

Like all large-scale social endeavors, there was a distance between the ideal and the actual. Mental illness proved protean and often intractable. The new asylums had trouble living up to their lofty goals, especially since they were mostly denied the level of resources needed to reach so high. Northampton was lucky to have one of the best of the new mental doctors running its hospital from early in its history until the mid-1880s. Pliny Earle, as much as any other person, was committed to the humane vision that animated the movement. He made this hospital a model of its kind. At the same time, his landmark studies showed that the hospitals were not curing most people, and that the nature and duration of the malady were most important in projecting future successful restoration to life outside.

Northampton began to exceed its intended capacity nearly as soon as it opened. Like every other hospital of its kind, it was always racing to find space for more beds. In times of social dislocation, it was a place to send people with all sorts of problems, not only people with a severe mental illness. The hospital was there and available, and its front door was always open. Perhaps, the most critical factor was the rise in the number of elderly people needing care. As early as the 1890s, ten percent of people being admitted were elderly. As life spans lengthened and local sources of assistance dwindled, the hospital accepted more and more old folks. By the mid-20th century, half of the patients being admitted were elderly, some with dementia or other mental maladies but many with only the typical needs for assistance with daily living. That type of need requires care, not treatment. At the same time, Northampton continued to be the only state institution in western Massachusetts to treat those with serious mental illness.

Pliny Earle would have been distressed by what he saw if he came back for a visit in 1950. There was now 10 times the original number of patients in residence at Northampton. The original buildings were still there, of course, but had been doubled by the construction of four additional wings, and five more large patient care structures had been added across Prince Street. Even so, patients were shoehorned in to every available space. People were still entering the hospital with acute episodes of illness, and some were recovering enough to leave again. But more were now finding the place a dead end. Instead of being visited by the superintendent every day, some went years without seeing or speaking to a doctor. The trappings of the moral therapy Earle championed were evident, but they were overwhelmed by the basic requirements of keeping in custody so many people with so many different needs.

Things changed in some very important ways in the last 65 years. A sea change in attitudes about individual rights and liberties has been translated into a range of new public policies. The nation took responsibility for the appalling need of so many of its elderly and created Medicare, making it possible to care for them outside the state hospitals. A movement to create places and programs in the community to assist people with severe mental illness has fundamentally changed their options. They can now choose different kinds of treatment, or they can choose none at all. The utopian project of 150 years ago to provide a place of asylum from the troubled world has been replaced by a different utopian project to create a society accepting of all people, even those with serious mental illness. Like the earlier project, this one has been tempered by real-world conditions and has its successes as well as failures. The extent to which our jails and prisons are filled with the mentally ill are a strong admonishment of our need to try harder.

Over the years, more than 65,000 people entered Northampton State Hospital and had the doors lock behind them. For every one of them, this was a life-changing event. Each time, this was done in our name. We have a responsibility to acknowledge this and to explore its meaning. This book of photographs is offered in that spirit. The images can only hint at the lived experience. The accompanying captions provide context. Wherever possible, the experience of those who walked through the door—and who too often never walked back out—is the focus.

One

Creation

The State Lunatic Hospital was consecrated at Northampton with much fanfare on the Fourth of July, 1856. There was cause to celebrate. The building, on a scale that dwarfed any other structure in the vicinity, proclaimed a large intention. This asylum was the fruit of a religiously inspired movement to treat people suffering from mental illness with kindness and caring. The large, central rotunda and corbeled gables of the massive building demonstrated the intention to provide substantial and sustained help for them.

Northampton lured Pliny Earle to the scene as its superintendent, a role he filled from 1864 to 1885. He was among the founders of the discipline of psychiatry in America, a discipline intimately wed to treatment in hospitals like Northampton. Under his leadership, the hospital provided humane care and an environment intended to ease disturbed minds and spirits and provide useful work and engaging recreation. From the start, there were too many patients for the size of the facility, which was filled virtually overnight by the transfer of patients from the state hospitals in Worcester and Taunton and from Boston City Hospital. Many had been disturbed for long periods of time, which reduced the ability of the staff in Northampton to help them get better.

Under Earle's tenure, the hospital became known for the extent to which work became an important aspect of therapy. The employment of patients on the farm, in the fields, and on the wards was seen as a central part of restoring them to health. Incidentally, it also served to reduce the costs of running a hospital that was regularly starved for financial support from the state. By carefully studying his own patients and the reports from other hospitals, Earle showed that the hospitals were not able to cure large numbers of patients, even if they did often ameliorate their distress. While superintendent, Earle unsuccessfully petitioned the state to change the name of the hospital to the Northampton Insane Hospital. The name was changed in 1899, and in 1905, it became Northampton State Hospital.

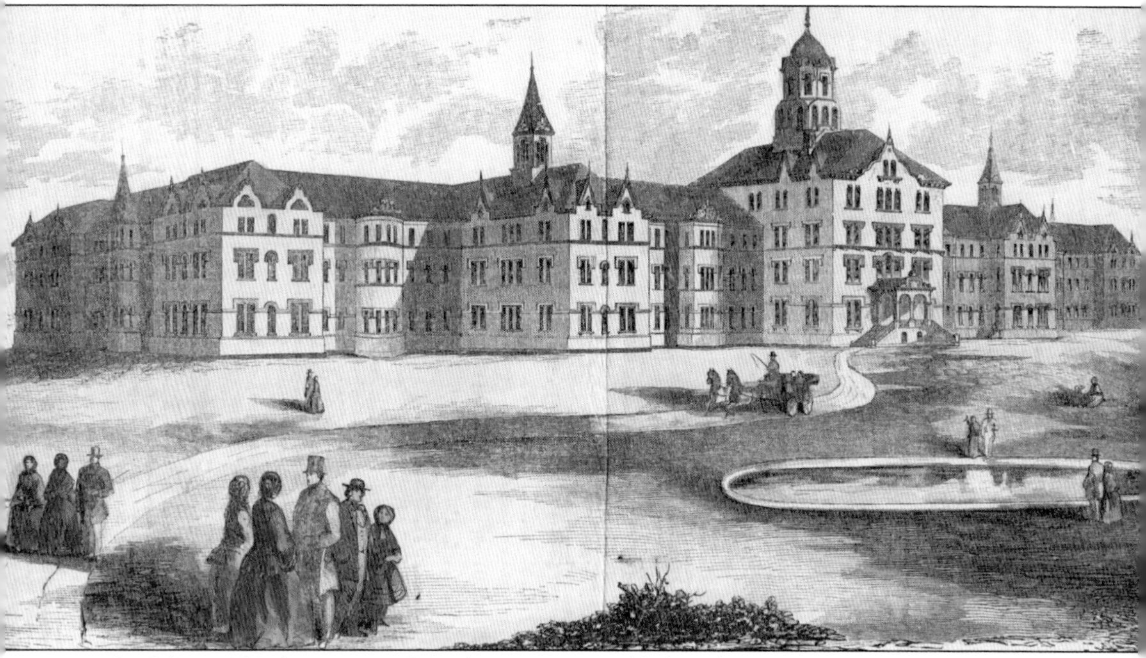

On July 4, 1856, the citizens of Northampton assembled on the occasion of laying the cornerstone of Northampton State Hospital. In the featured address, Edward Jarvis said the following: "It is the especial duty of the Commonwealth to heal the wounds it inflicts or allows to be inflicted and to provide the means of curing and protecting the insane. . . . They saw that there was a need of more Hospitals and they therefore determined to erect this Hospital. . . . You then, you the people, have duties as well as the State, and these obligations will rest upon you, as long as the Hospital shall endure, or as long as you and your children and your children's children shall be subject to the terrible diseases which this house is established to cure or alleviate. . . . You of this town and the counties can and will do much for the prosperity and the comfort of this new Institution, and then this Hospital will ever have reason to rejoice, that it is placed in the midst of an enlightened and a generous community."

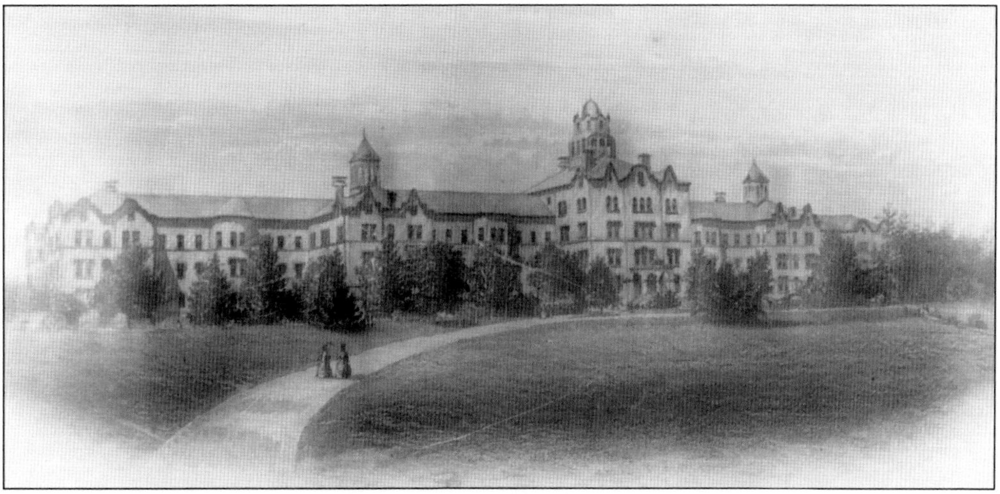

The original facade spanned 519 feet and extended across 9 wards on each side, 18 in all. The two sides of the building were seen as completely separate and were described as follows: "The keys for the male and female wards should be so entirely different that it will be impossible to make those for one side open the locks for the other. Male attendants should never be allowed to go into a female ward, which would be conclusive proof of a most defective discipline," according to influential hospital designer Thomas Kirkbride.

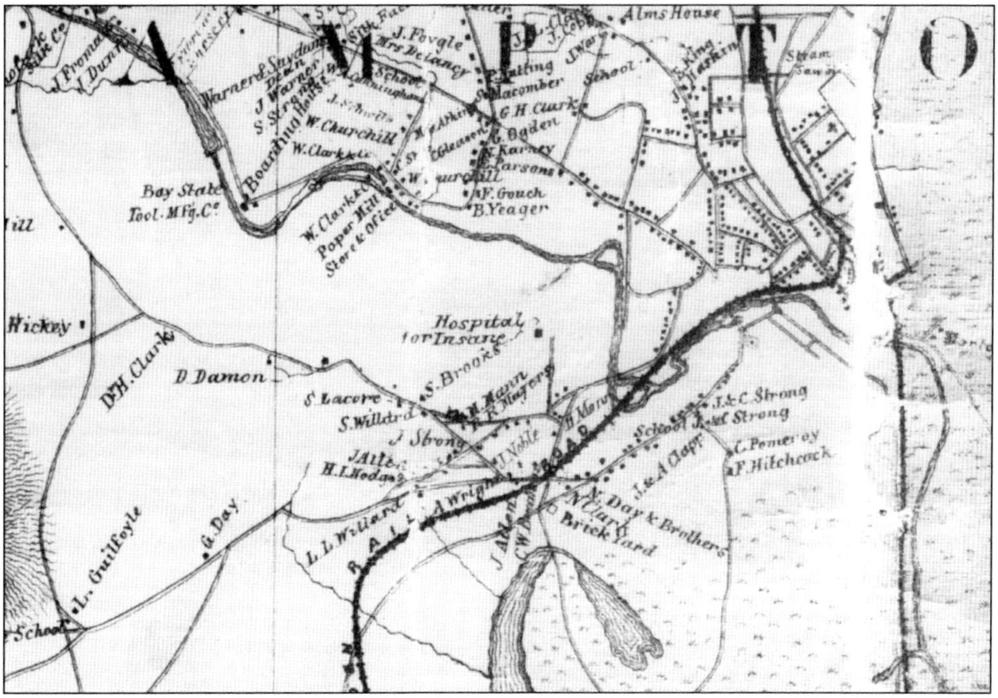

Shown is a detail from an 1860 wall map of Hampshire County. It designates the hospital as "Hospital for Insane." Similar 19th-century maps listed the hospital as "Northampton Lunatic Hospital." Naturally bordered by Northampton's Mill River and Paradise Pond, the hospital was situated on a magnificent slope facing south and west. Smith College (1875) became its immediate neighbor, the two institutions eventually comprising Northampton's largest employers. In 1860, the hospital was serving a total of 434 patients, with 104 admissions and 30 deaths.

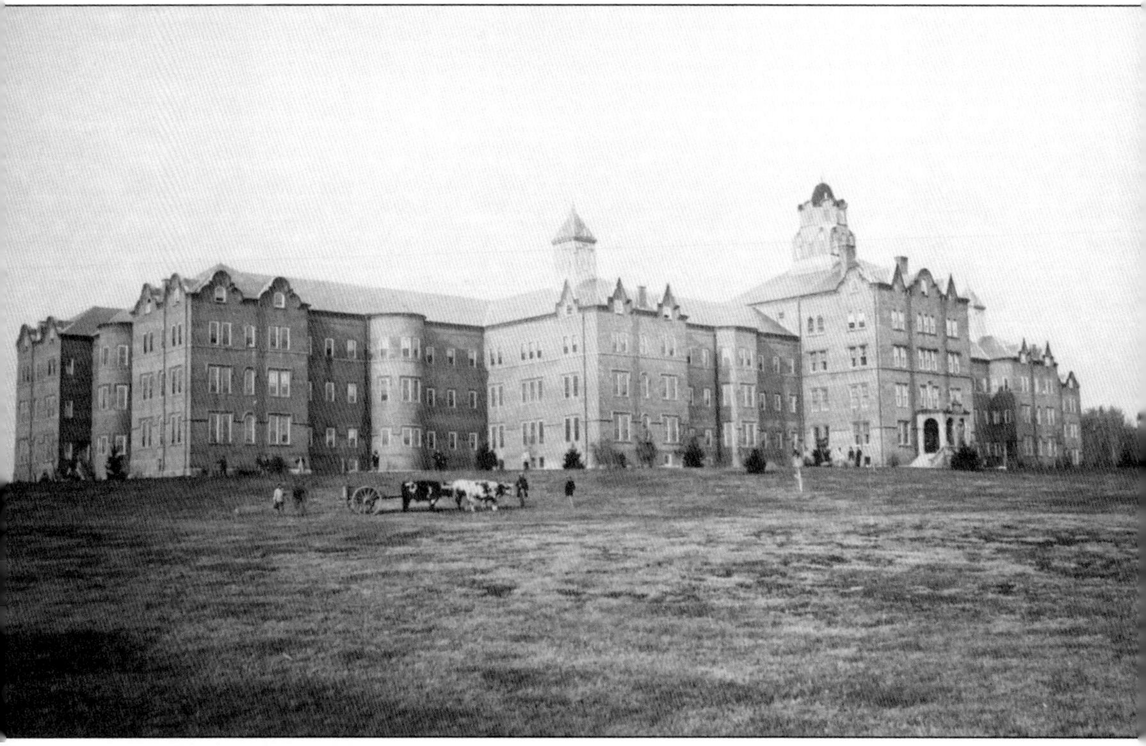

Northampton State Hospital was designed by Jonathan Preston of Boston (1801–1888). This rare style, with its steep roof gables, was described as Elizabethan when new but is now referred to as Jacobean. It also featured Italianate pedimented and Serlian windows, a cupola, and angled bay windows. The symmetrical layout, shown here in its opening year of 1858, which has stepped-back wings for female patients on the left side and male patients on the right, was built in accordance with the treatise "On the Construction, Organization, and General arrangements of Hospitals for the Insane" by Thomas Kirkbride. For almost four decades, this influential guide was used throughout the United States, resulting in more than 50 "Kirkbride" institutions. These hospitals were not to exceed a capacity of 250 patients, a directive that proved untenable as admissions rose steadily over the decades. Most of the original Kirkbride hospitals, Northampton State Hospital included, grew to accommodate 10 times as many patients as had been recommended.

These brownstone entry gates stood sentinel at the main entrance to Northampton State Hospital for nearly its entire history, framing the central building and its imposing rotunda. The wrought iron fence extends from here in both directions to a total length of well over a mile, enclosing the hospital and its hundreds of acres of farm and fields.

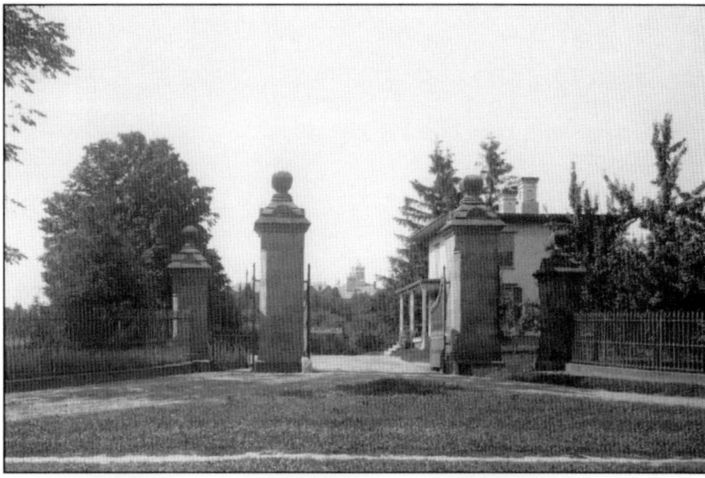

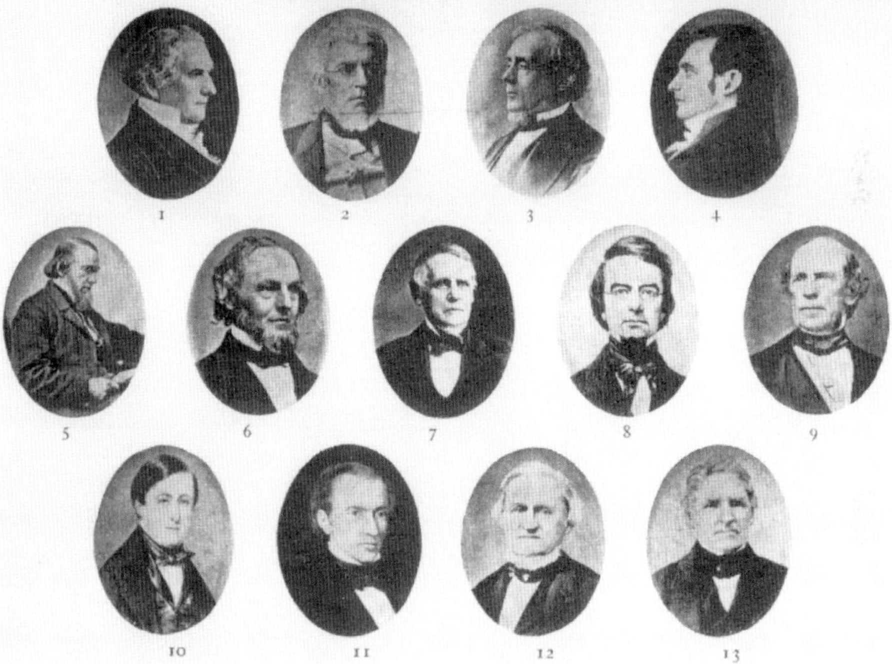

THE ORIGINAL THIRTEEN

(1) Samuel B. Woodward, (2) Isaac Ray, (3) John S. Butler, (4) Samuel White, (5) Charles H. Stedman, (6) Pliny Earle, (7) Thomas S. Kirkbride, (8) Luther V. Bell, (9) William L. Awl, (10) John M. Galt, (11) Amariah Brigham, (12) Francis T. Stribling, (13) Nehemiah Cutter.

When 25 mental hospitals had already been established in the United States, the Association of Medical Superintendents of American Institutions for the Insane (AMSAII) was founded in Philadelphia in 1844 at a meeting of 13 superintendents. Pliny Earle was one of the founders. It was the first professional medical specialty organization in the country. The objectives of the association were "to communicate their experiences to each other, cooperate in collecting statistical information relating to insanity, and assist each other in improving the treatment of the insane," according to the US Library of Medicine. In 1921, the name was changed to the present American Psychiatric Association.

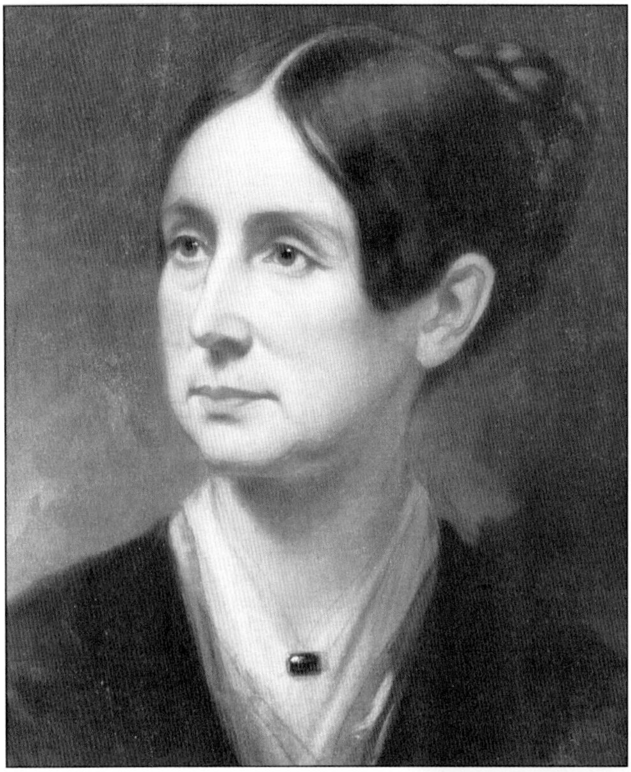

"I tell what I have seen . . . painful and shocking," Dorothea Dix wrote in her groundbreaking "Memorial to the Legislature of Massachusetts" in 1843. Dorothea Dix (1802–1887) was a remarkable whistleblower and social reformer, working tirelessly together with legislators, politicians, and presidents on improving the care for the mentally ill and the disabled. A close friend and constant correspondent of Pliny Earle's who visited him in Northampton several times, Dix was instrumental in the founding of more than 30 psychiatric institutions in the United States. Samuel Waugh created this 1868 oil painting. (Courtesy of National Portrait Gallery, Smithsonian Institution; transfer from the St. Elizabeths Hospital Museum.)

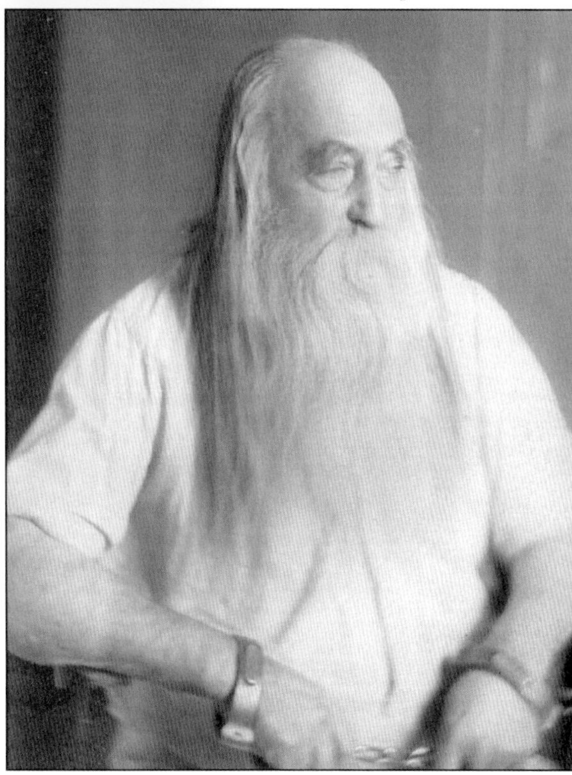

This photograph was long held in the archives of the hospital. It illustrates the fact that nearly all of the first patients admitted in 1858 were transferred from hospitals in Worcester and Boston and that some were shackled during the trip. In contrast, the superintendent reported in the second month the hospital was open, "We have been enabled thus far to dispense with the use of all means of personal restraint, no apparatus of any kind having as yet been used upon any patient." This man is unidentified.

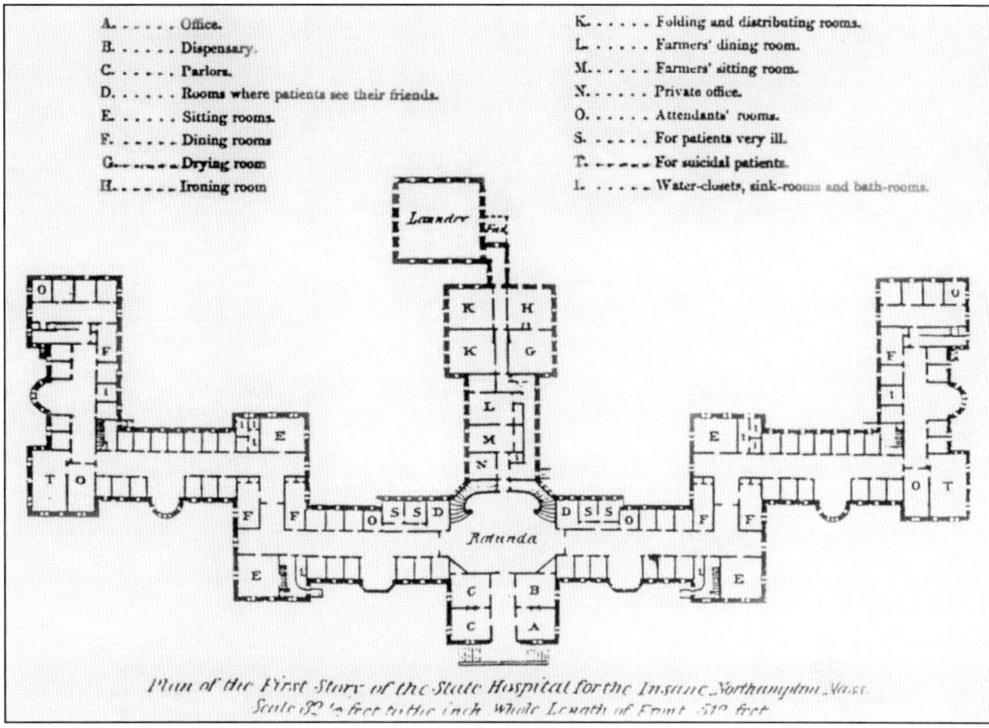

Northampton State Hospital was the third state hospital built in Massachusetts, after Worcester (1832) and Taunton (1851). Based on the idea of moral treatment, it was designed as a single, massive building with the superintendent at its center and symmetrical wings on each side "as to give ample accommodations for the resident officers and their families and for the classification and comfort of the patients," wrote Thomas Kirkbride.

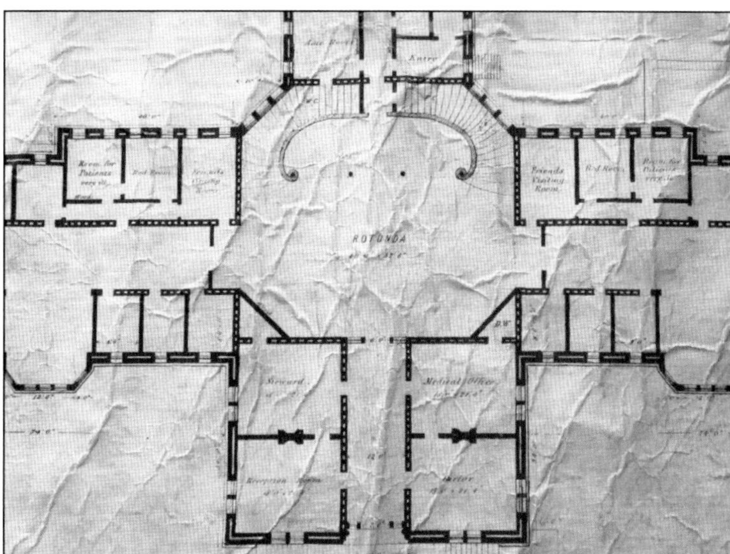

In the center were located the superintendent's office, parlors, the farmers' dining and sitting rooms, the chapel, and the apartments for the superintending physician's family. Perhaps most notable about the original layout is the inclusion of a friends visiting room, hinting at the hospital's early emphasis on enabling the relationship of its patients with the community at large.

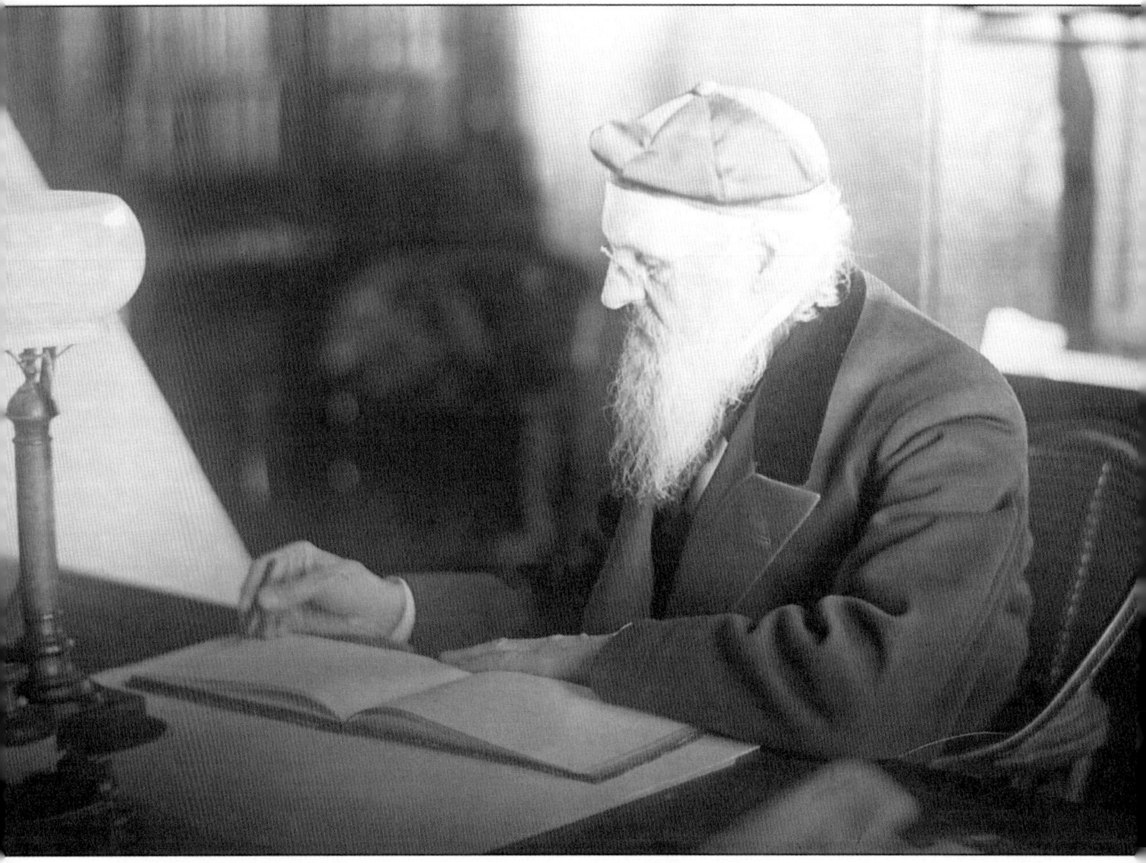

Pliny Earle (1809–1892) came to Northampton a worldly and experienced practitioner of the art of healing. He had studied the treatment of the mentally ill in Europe and America and had worked as a doctor in famous hospitals in Philadelphia and New York. He epitomized the ideal of the superintendent. No detail of the hospital and its operation was too small for his attention, and everything was to conduce to creating a therapeutic world for his ill charges. He was humane and compassionate. Treating his patients as complete human beings, he created chances for them to dance, pray, work, learn, and think about the world and about their own condition. Even so, he was clear-eyed about the limits of his impact on their health. Using careful analysis, he demonstrated that the utopian claims for high rates of cure made by the asylum builders did not stand up to close scrutiny. He ran the hospital for 20 years and lived out his retirement in his apartments there. He bequeathed large sums to Northampton for its library and for the care of its elderly poor. He is buried in Bridge Street Cemetery in Northampton.

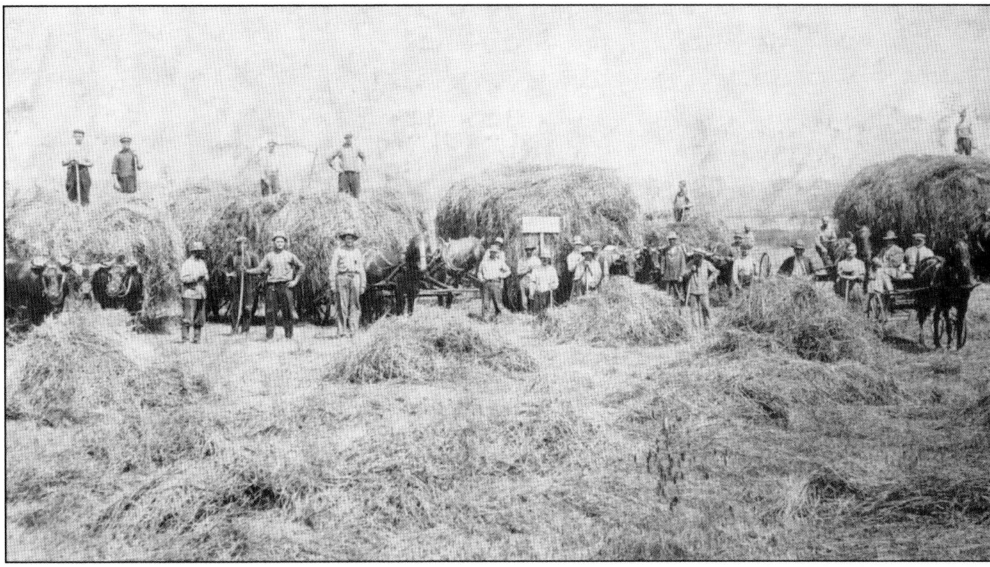

A farm was purchased as the site for the hospital, and patients worked on it from its first year of operation. "The value of the crops is by no means the measure of the value of the farm to the institution. By constant and regular exercise on the farm . . . disordered trains of thought, and morbid states of feeling are interrupted, and a healthy interest in surrounding objects excited and maintained," wrote the superintendent in the 1858 annual report.

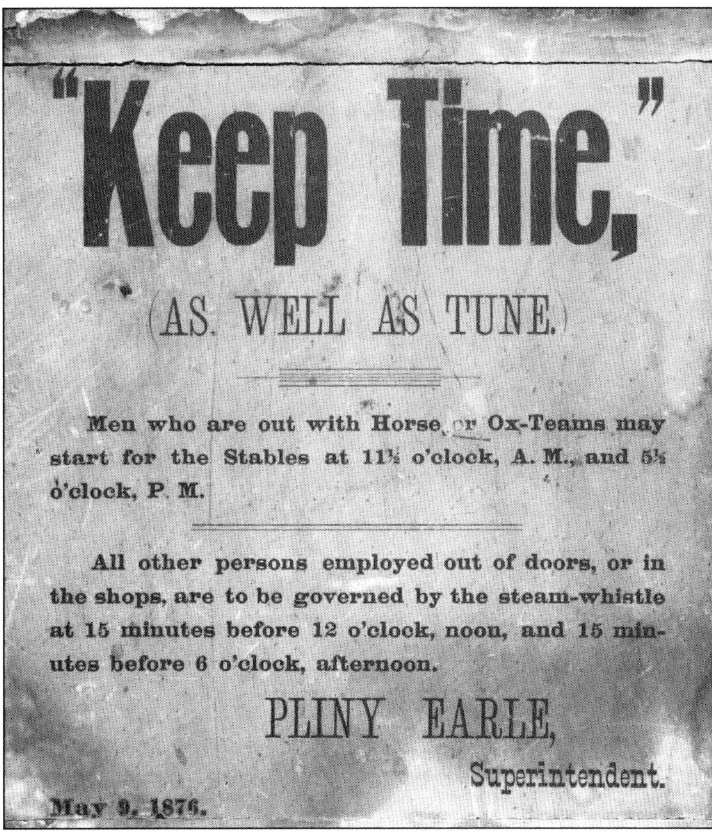

"Keep Time,"

(AS WELL AS TUNE.)

Men who are out with Horse or Ox-Teams may start for the Stables at 11½ o'clock, A. M., and 5½ o'clock, P. M.

All other persons employed out of doors, or in the shops, are to be governed by the steam-whistle at 15 minutes before 12 o'clock, noon, and 15 minutes before 6 o'clock, afternoon.

PLINY EARLE,

Superintendent.

May 9, 1876.

"Believing a call for general action would promote punctuality, order and systematic working, a steam-whistle was placed above the engine-house and connected with one of the boilers; and since that time has been regularly used," wrote Pliny Earle. In his 21 years of serving as superintendent, Earle doubled the hospital's acreage and vastly increased crop yields, from 40 tons of hay and 6,256 pounds of pork in 1864 to 251 tons of hay and 17,544 pounds of pork in 1885.

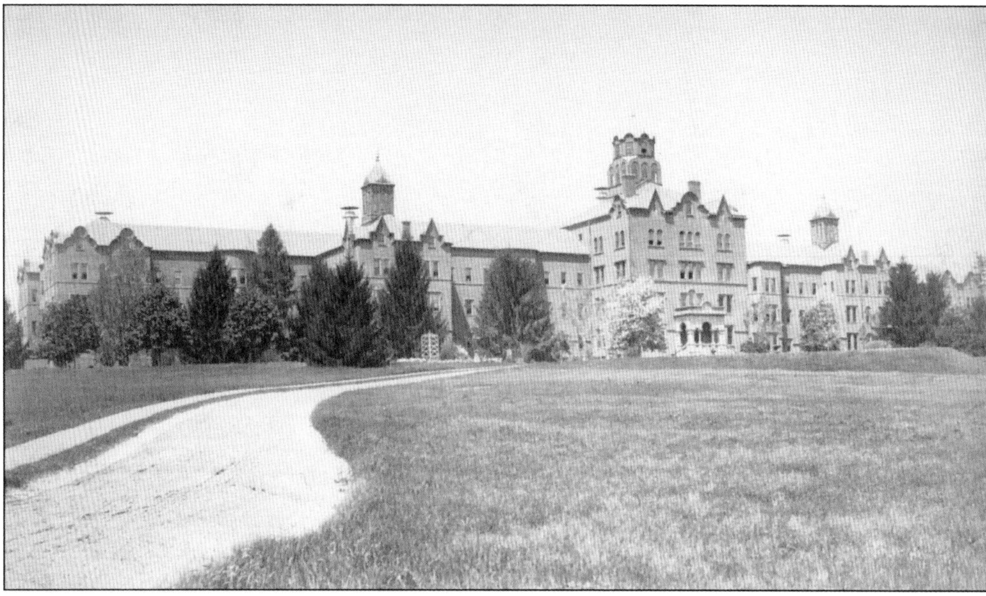

The hospital fulfilled its role as both a place of healing and a place of refuge in the 1870s and 1880s. The number of patients held steady in this period at about 450. Many people were admitted with acute mental symptoms, and many were discharged within a year, having been cured or stabilized enough to return to the community. About three in four admissions stayed more than a year at the hospital, but some stayed for significant lengths of time.

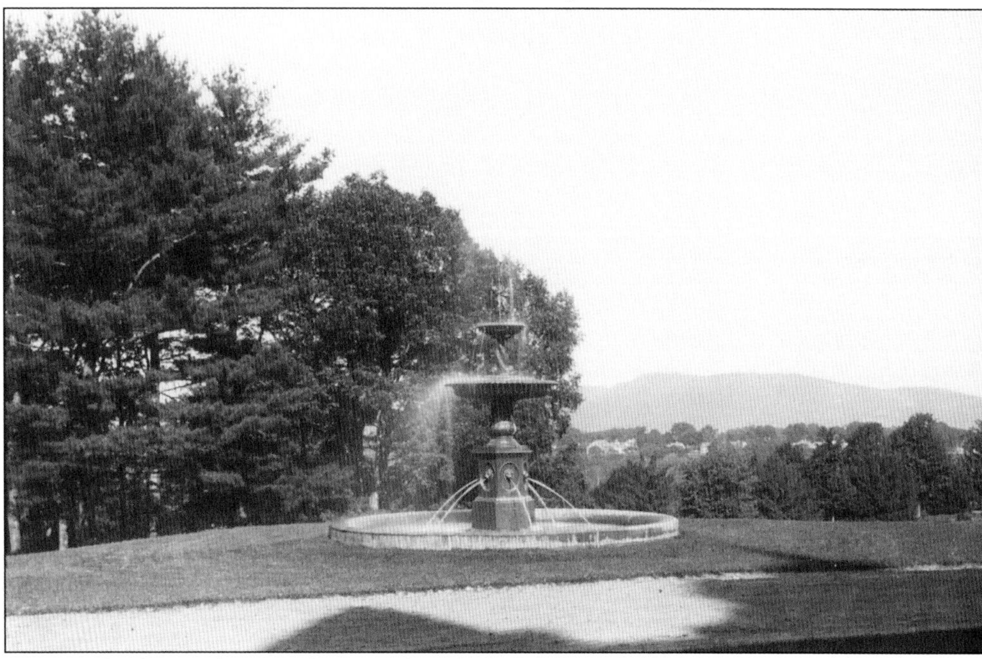

In 1876, the hospital's annual report described that an iron fountain was erected "directly in front of the central doorway, and at a distance from it of 121 feet. The ground basin is 16 feet in diameter, surrounded by a heavy curb of hewn granite. Fountain, curb, and basin are upon a superstructure of solid stone masonry six feet in height. The cost of the fountain was near $1,200."

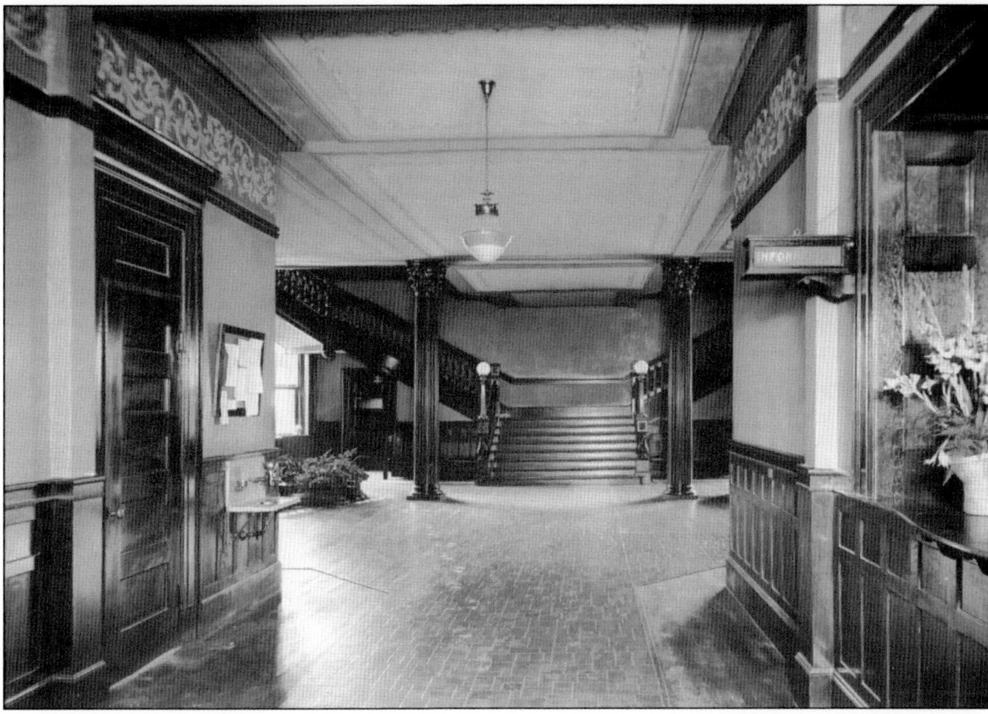

"The building should be in good taste, and it should impress favorably not only the patients, but their friends and others who may visit it. Nor is the influence of these things on the friends of patients unimportant; they cannot fail to see that neither labor nor expense is spared to promote the happiness of the patients, and they are thus led to have a generous confidence in those whose care their friends have been entrusted," wrote Thomas Kirkbride. This is the main entrance, the central rotunda, that a patient or visitor would have entered. Upstairs lived the superintendent until 1940, when a new house was constructed for him, and the old quarters were converted to a surgical suite and infirmary for sick employees. In 1958–1959, the rotunda was floored over on all three floors.

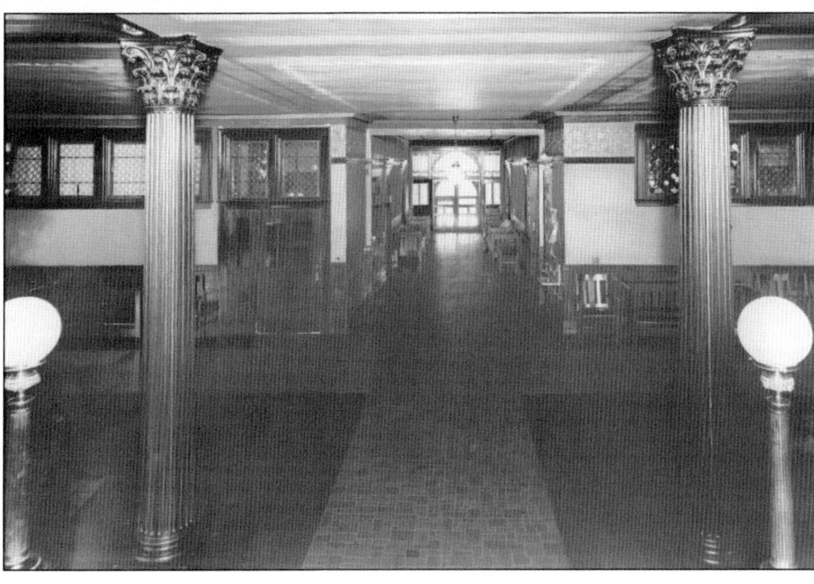

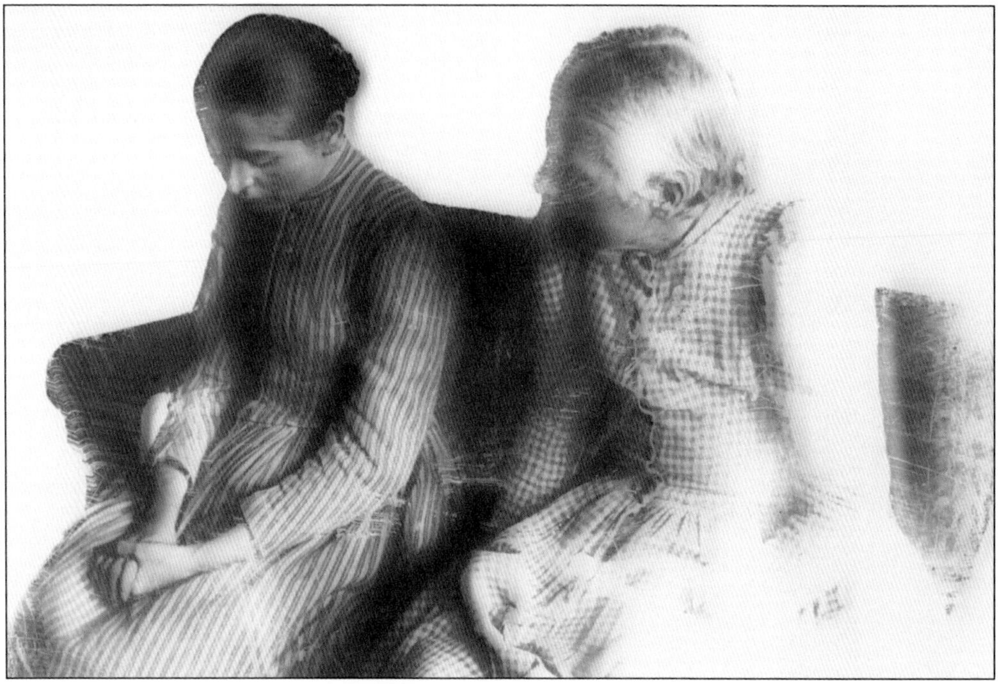

These three unidentified patients were probably photographed about 1900. That year, 242 people were admitted to the hospital. Among the women, the most common background was as a domestic or factory worker. This was true for the men as well; although, there were many farmers. Intemperance was considered the cause of illness for nearly one third of the men, while heredity or senility were considered most responsible for the travails of the women. The year 1900 was a particularly bad year for disease at the hospital. Typhoid fever ravaged the staff and patients from September to November. Two nurses and eight patients died. It was suspected that the source of the disease was celery raised on the hospital farm. The hospital's pleas for help were answered when the infirmary wards were built over the next five years.

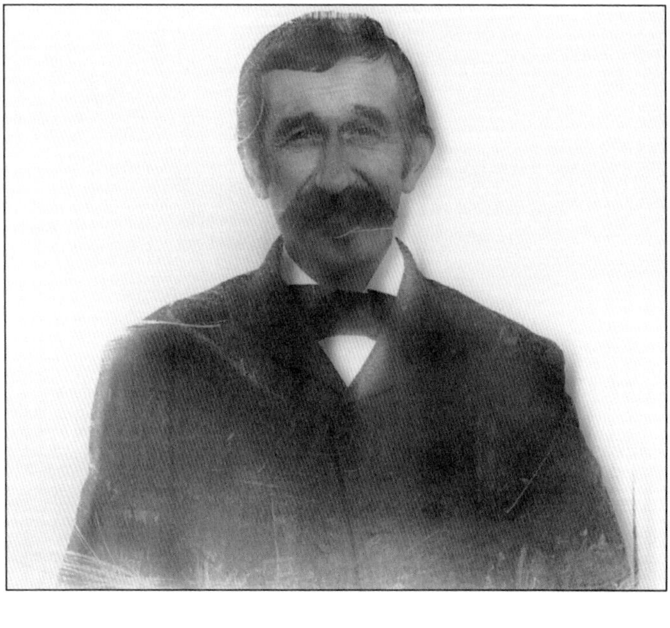

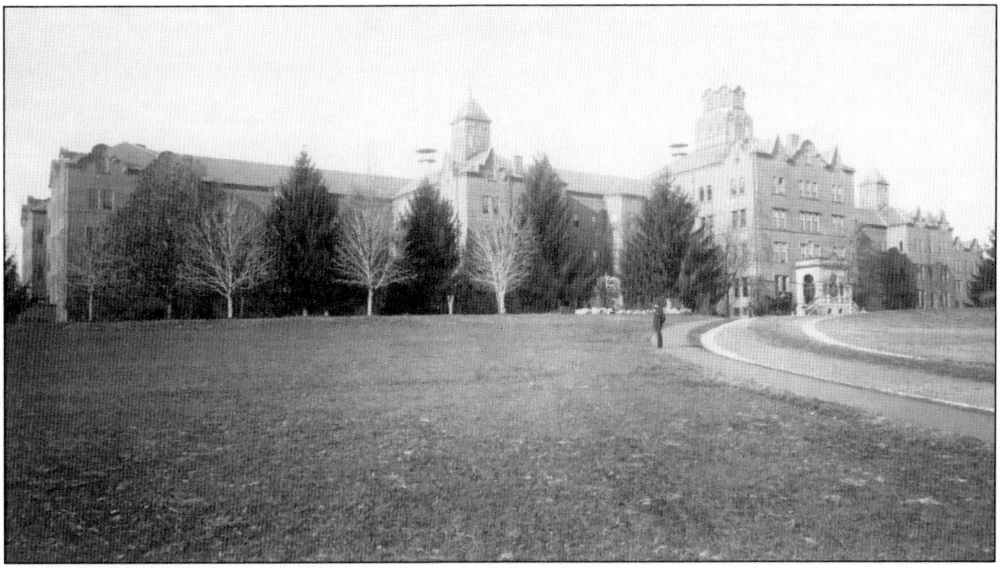

As patient numbers continued to outgrow the architecture, the trustees wrote the following in 1885: "Twenty-inch brick walls do not readily yield to internal pressure, and when the enclosed room has received a proper and wholesome number of inmates, every additional occupant is an encroachment upon the convenience, the comfort, and the health of the whole."

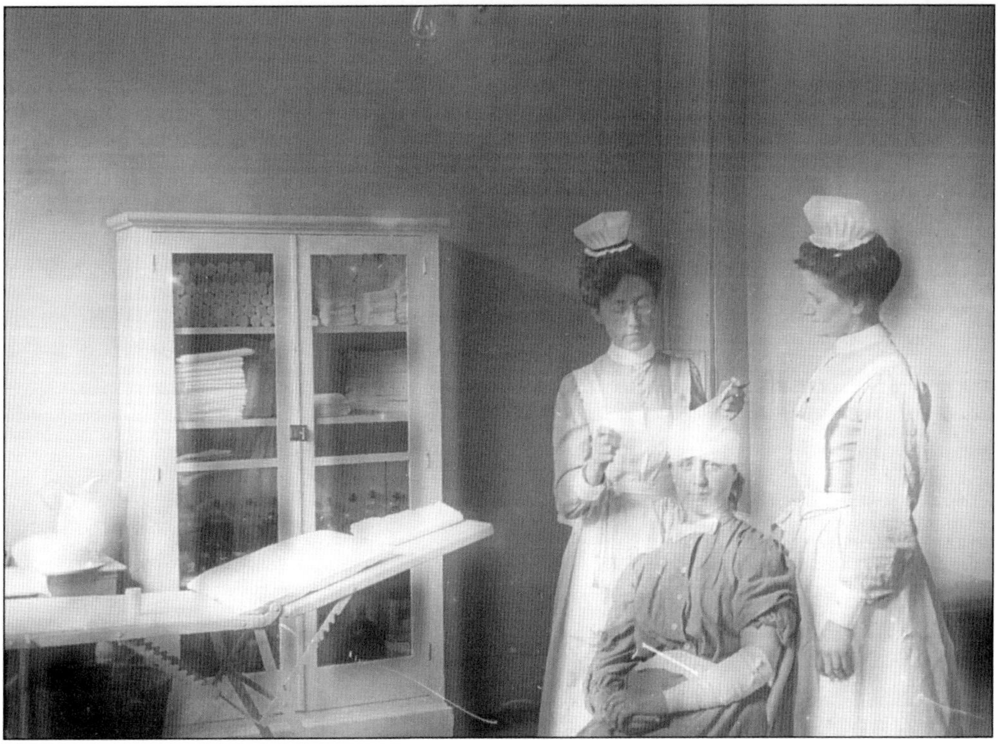

A nurse in training receives instruction in applying first aide in this glass print from around 1900. A training program was established in 1898. In the 1920s, students began to spend time studying at general hospitals in Holyoke and in Tewksbury. In 1935, a two-year course in psychiatric nursing was established but was discontinued during World War II.

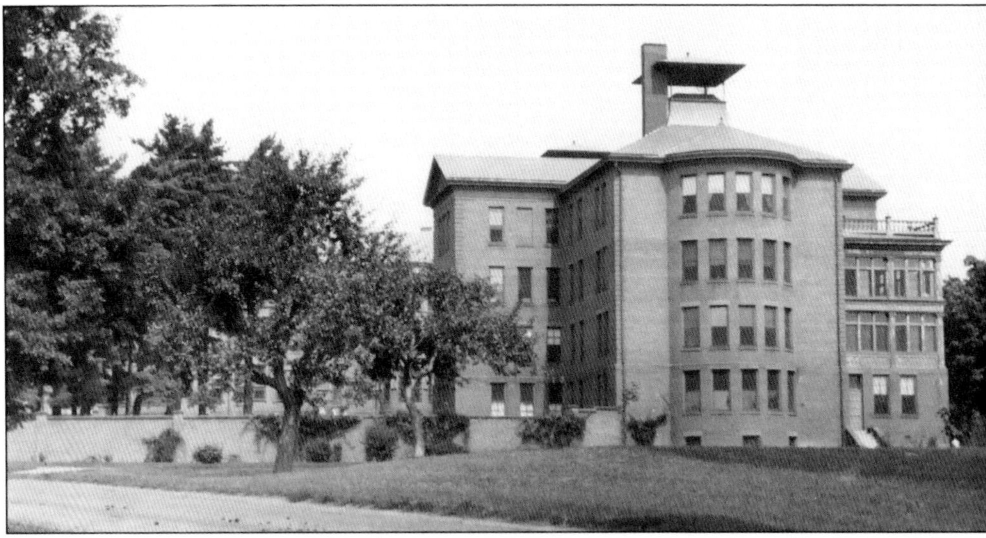

The South Infirmary was completed in 1903 as the place to care for physically ill or frail female patients. The new facility would help isolate those with contagious diseases and ease the terrible overcrowding on the wards. When new, it housed 70 patients, as well as 20 nurses, who were relocated from rooms on the old wards. The airing court walls, constructed in 1872, are visible on the left.

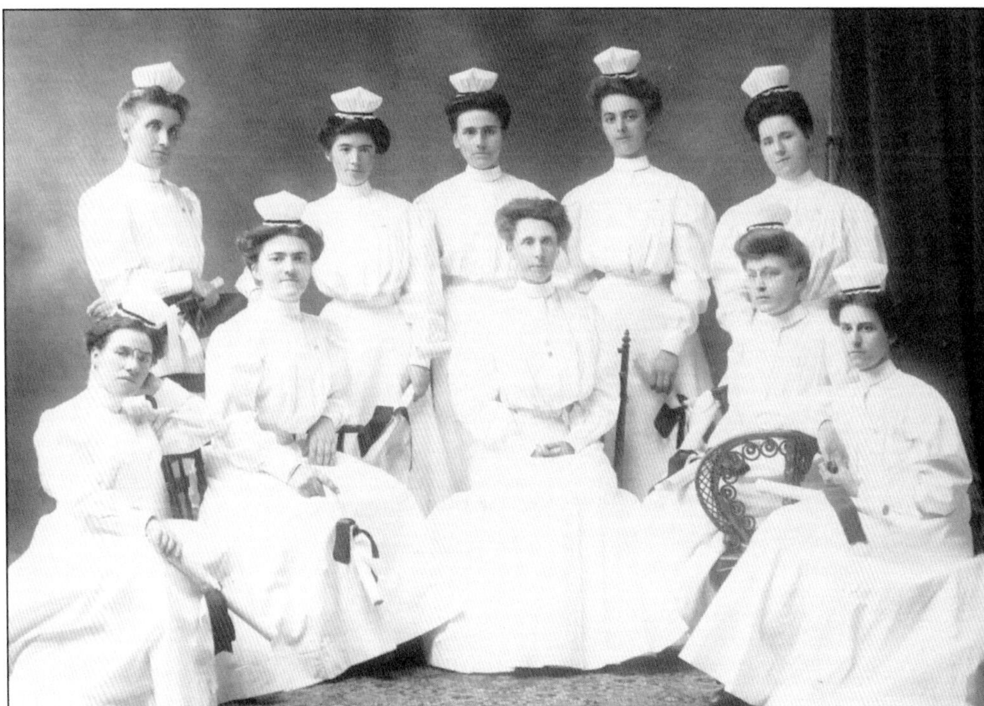

The nurses' training program was designed to improve the quality of care and to make the hospital a more appealing place to work. However, none of these 1907 graduates was still working at the hospital five years after graduation. Professional training was a way out of the low pay and difficult working conditions of the state hospital.

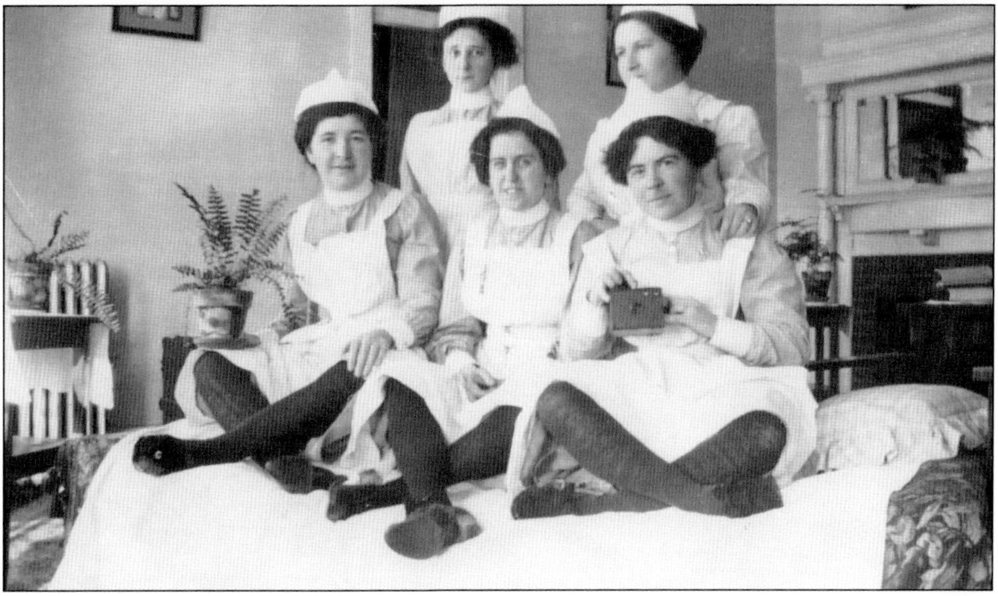

The small size of this nursing school class of 1915 is typical of the period. According to the superintendent, "There is such great demand for pupil nurses in general hospitals everywhere that young women with a sincere desire for training have no difficulty in finding places open to them in general hospitals, the nature of our service making State hospitals second choice." The nurse with the camera is Sarah Mary Sharpe, known as Sadie.

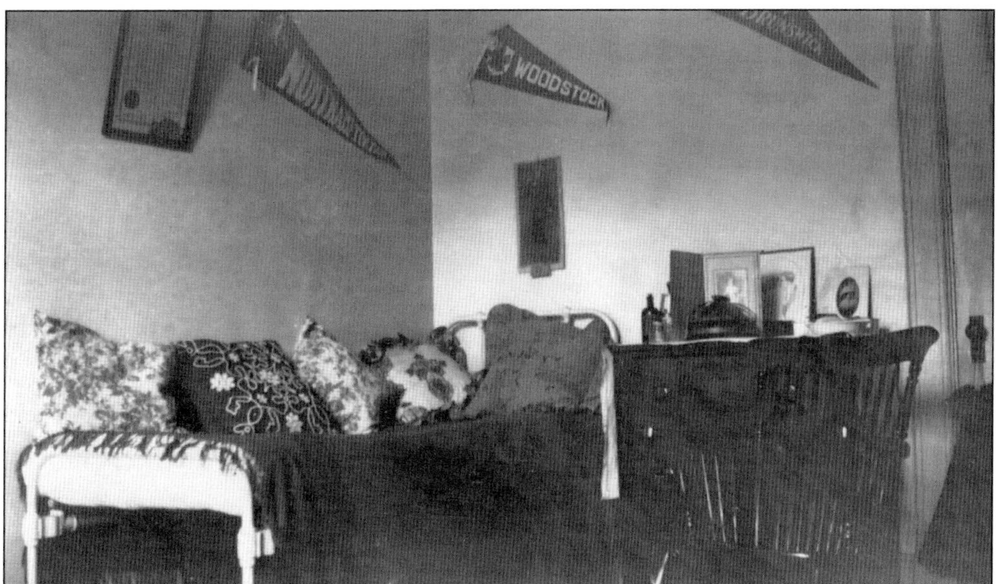

Looking much like a college dormitory, this is the room of Sarah Sharpe on the top floor of the South Infirmary about 1915. Sharpe was a student in the nurses training program and subsequently had a long career at the hospital.

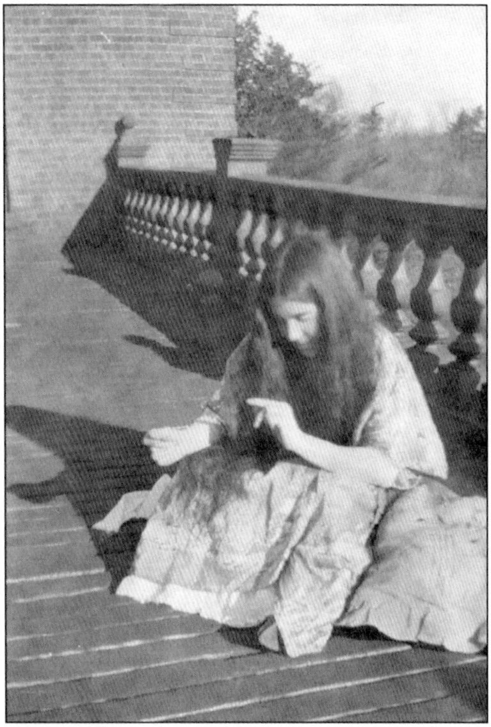

This unusually intimate and private photograph of Sarah Sharpe hints at the complex lives of people who both worked and lived at the hospital. This 1915 picture was taken on the balcony on the top floor of the South Infirmary. The last worker apartment in the Nurses' Home was not shuttered until 1984.

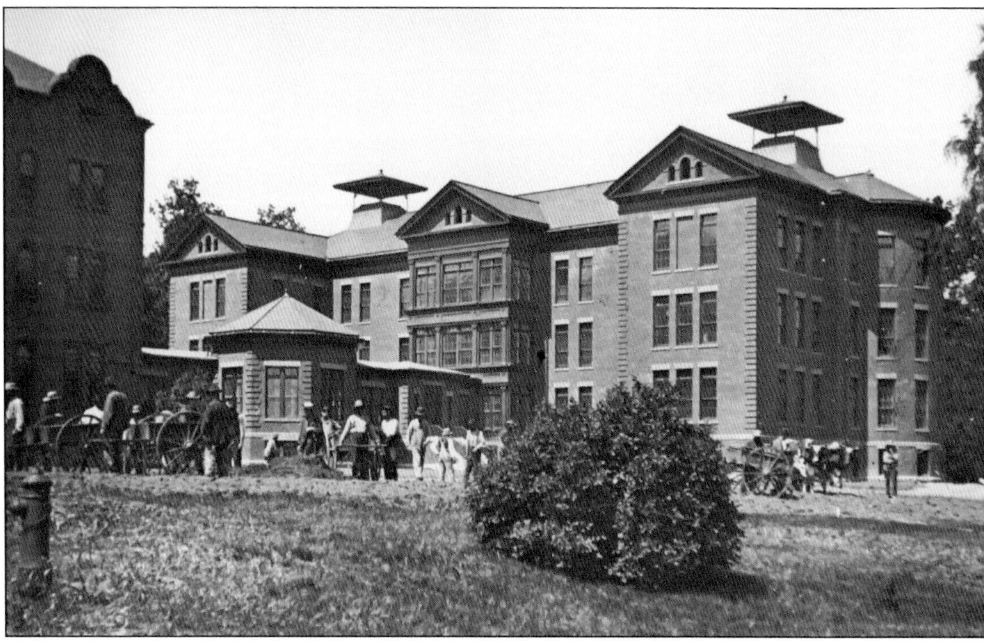

"Planned so that every room occupied by patients gets sunshine," the men's infirmary was built for 100 patients and 34 nurses and was completed in 1905, stated the hospital's annual report. It was located about 100 feet north of the north wing, "far enough away to permit unobstructed light and air," and was connected to the main building by a one-story corridor with an octagonal sun room. In 1937, the wooden floors were replaced with concrete ones, and an enclosed staircase was added as further means of fireproofing.

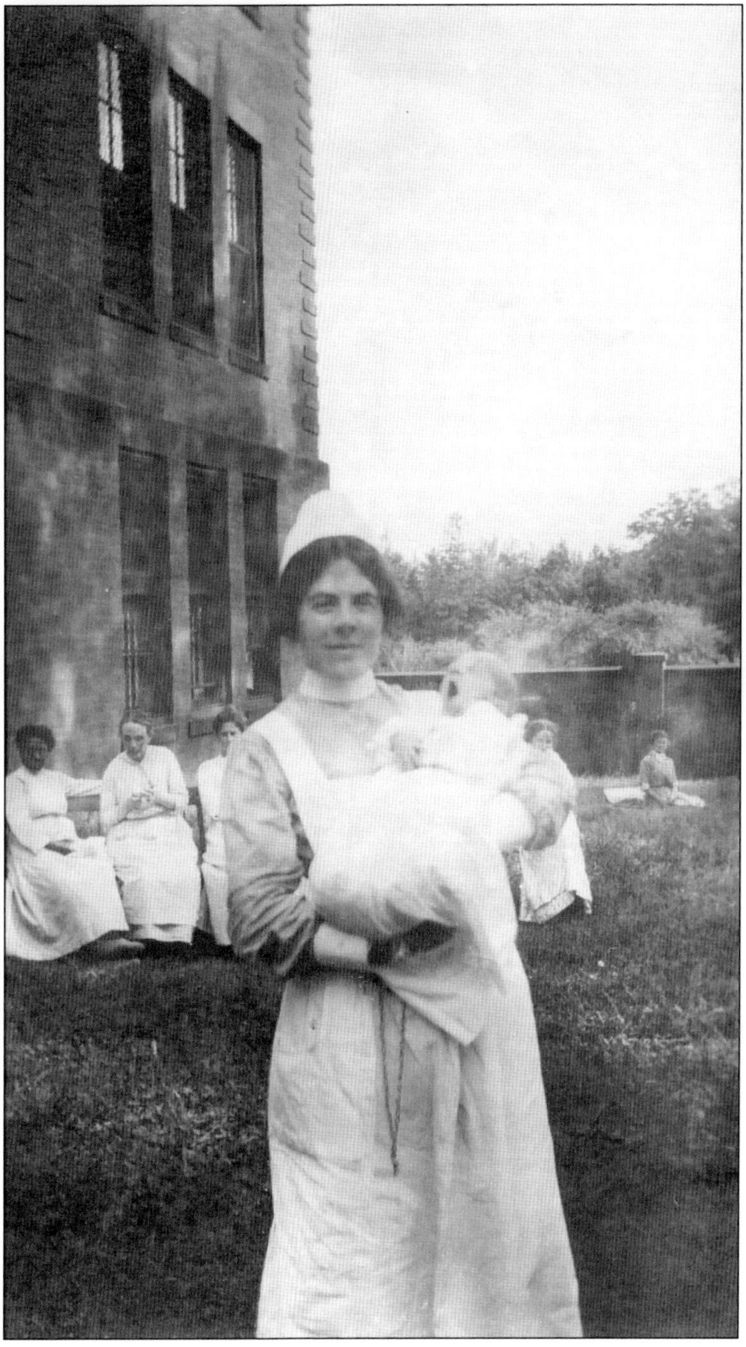

Nurse Sarah Sharpe holds a baby while standing in the airing court on the south side of the hospital in this richly detailed photograph. Several unidentified patients sit behind her. It is extremely rare to see a baby in this setting, and no information is available about the child. Possibly, it is the child of a former employee come back to visit. Perhaps, the mother is a patient. In this period, a woman who became pregnant outside of marriage had few sources of support for herself or her child. Unwed mothers were often treated as feebleminded or degenerate. Perhaps, the mother found the hospital the only available place for care.

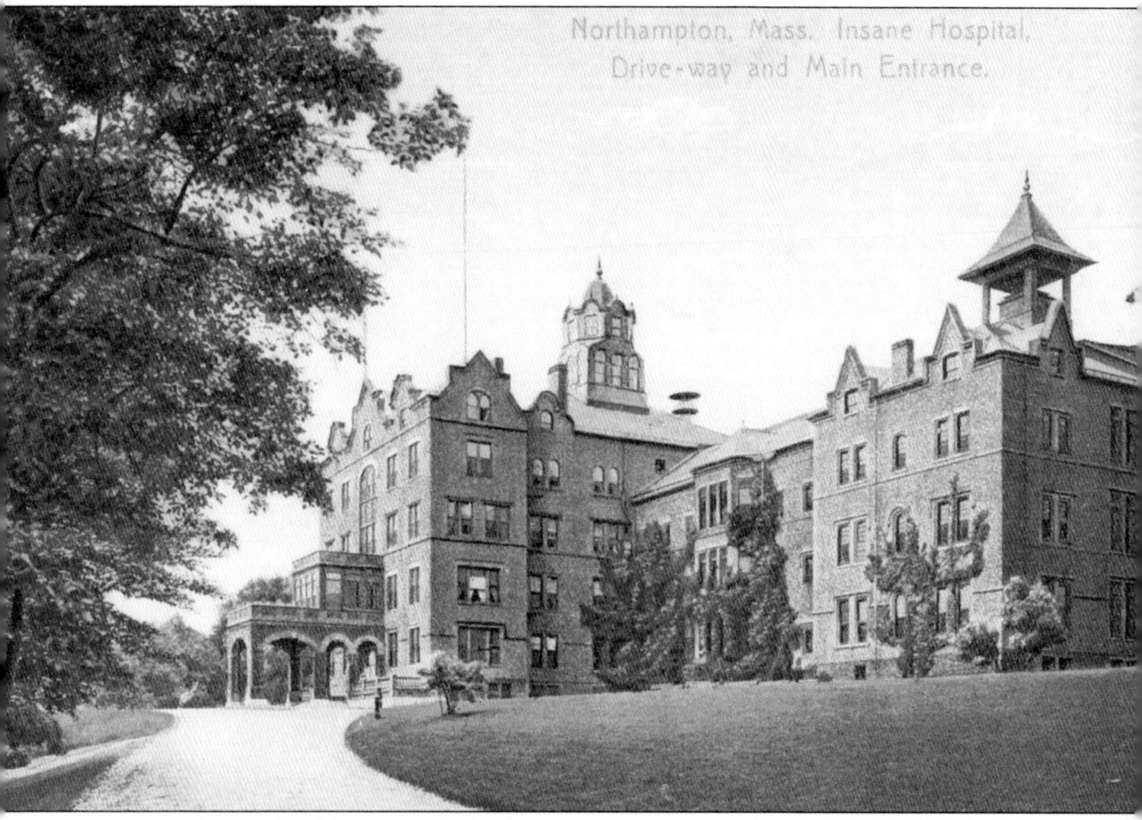

The northern side of the hospital's driveway loop is shown in this colored postcard, looking up at the front entrance of the hospital. The front was remodeled in 1899, adding a four-story addition, three bays deep and five bays wide, built with brick with brownstone trim. The 1877 portico was extended out two bays to form a porte cochere and an enclosed porch, where passengers might alight under cover. The ivy, which covered vast stretches of the main building in its later years, is beginning to crawl up the walls of the north side, and the dome is still in place, cutting an imposing silhouette against the west. A retired nurse remembered, "People in the community just thought that anyone who was up here was crazy and violent, and that just was not true. Our society at that time thought that if people are mentally ill, you put them away somewhere and forget about them. But there were other people. I remember on Friday nights the families would come and take their patients home, and back on Sunday night."

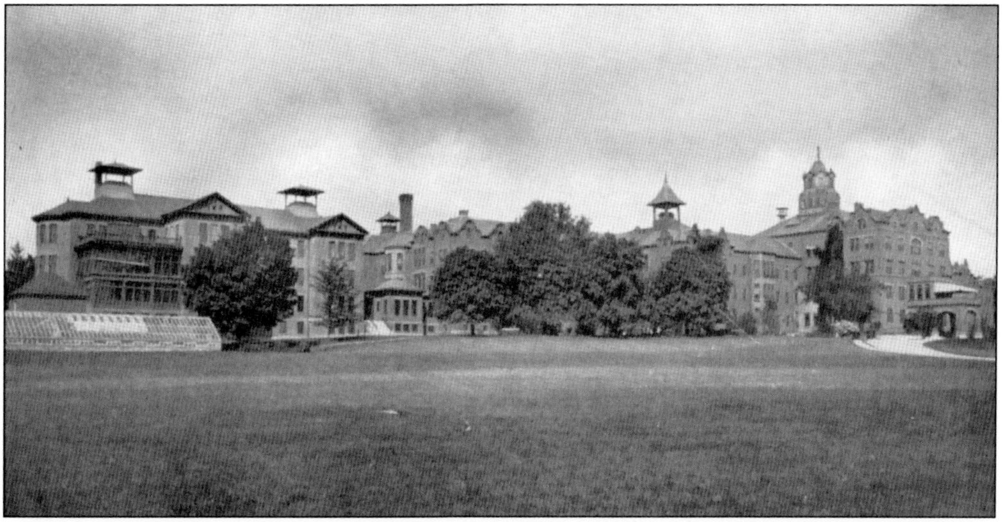

The original design propositions by Kirkbride included a strong caution against allowing hospitals to house more than 250 patients in a single building. As the average hospital size increased nonetheless, Kirkbride's influence declined. All around the country, hospitals were adding wings and additions—Northampton State Hospital included. Infirmaries were constructed here between 1903 and 1905 on either side of the main building, enlarging the original facade to more than 800 feet in total length.

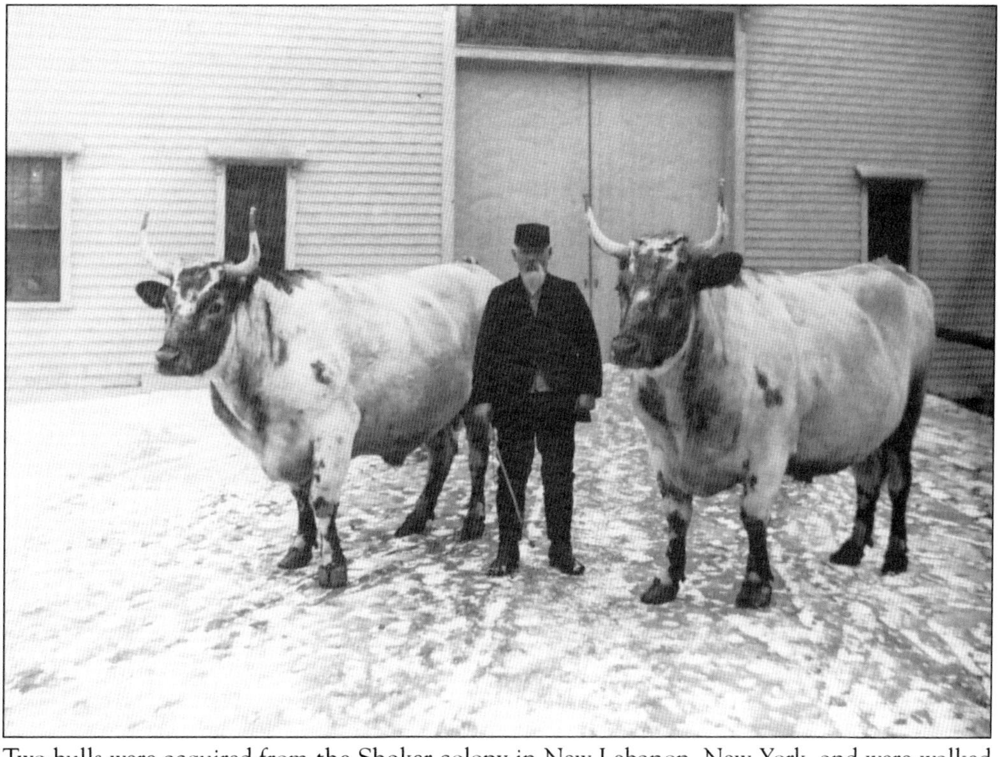

Two bulls were acquired from the Shaker colony in New Lebanon, New York, and were walked the 50 miles from there to the hospital in Northampton. The trek took two weeks. The bulls were named Sarcastic DeCall and Shaker Bull No. 2. The handler's name has not been identified.

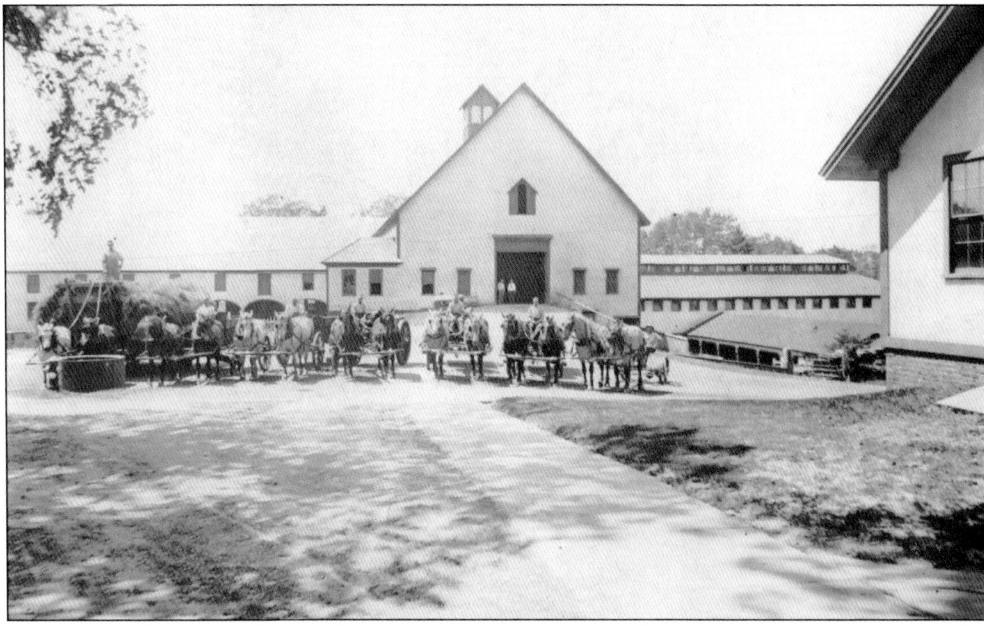

The extensions to this barn were added in 1901 to accommodate the large hospital milk herd. The two-story wing to the right housed 70 milk cows on its upper floor, with room for 70 steers below. The 1.5-story wing to the left was used for calves. A total of 68 cows produced more than 66,000 gallons of milk in 1918.

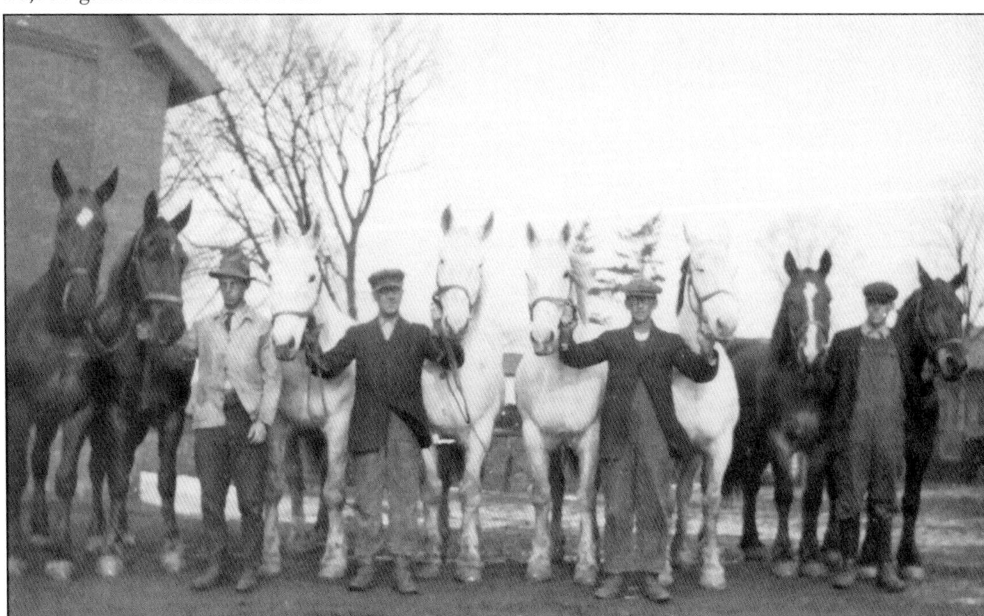

Before tractors replaced draft horses in agriculture, America had 26 million horses and mules at its all-time high in 1918. Farmhands had long-lasting relationships with their animals. For patients working on the farm, the animals were therapeutic. There were other benefits of farm work as well. "If he was a good worker, he had it made, he'll always have good shoes and boots. He never was without cigarettes. He could take a shower twice a week whether he needed it or not. He was one of the farm workers," remembers Sue Eaton, director of nurses.

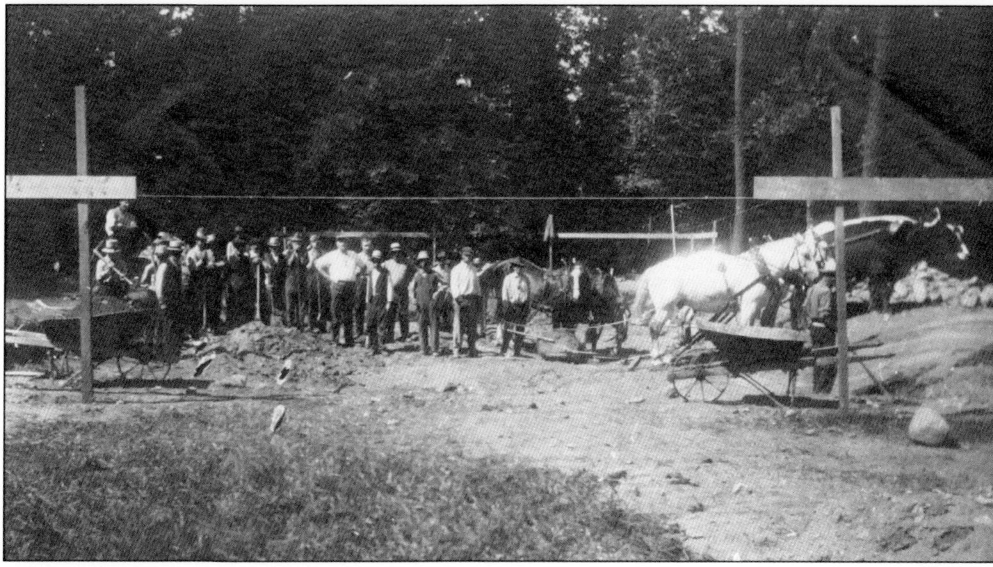

Patients comprise this construction crew supervised by hospital staff. They may be working to build a recreation pavilion for men in 1907. Patients had earlier helped to erect several other hospital buildings. The superintendent wrote, "Several of the patients who were thus employed have been discharged [as] recovered and many of them improved. Their interest in the work, the mental diversion and the benefit that comes from occupation contributed largely to these favorable results."

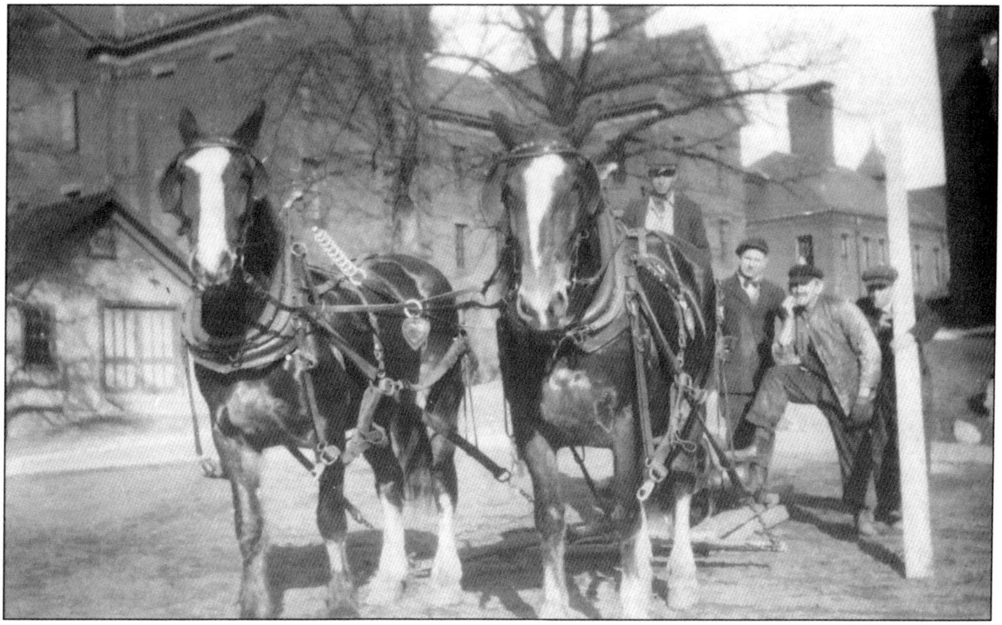

A group of hospital workers shows off a team of draft horses in this photograph from about 1915. Directly behind them is the dormitory established in 1892 for those male patients who were full-time workers on the farm. A total of 50 men lived in this converted building, which was very convenient to the barns and fields.

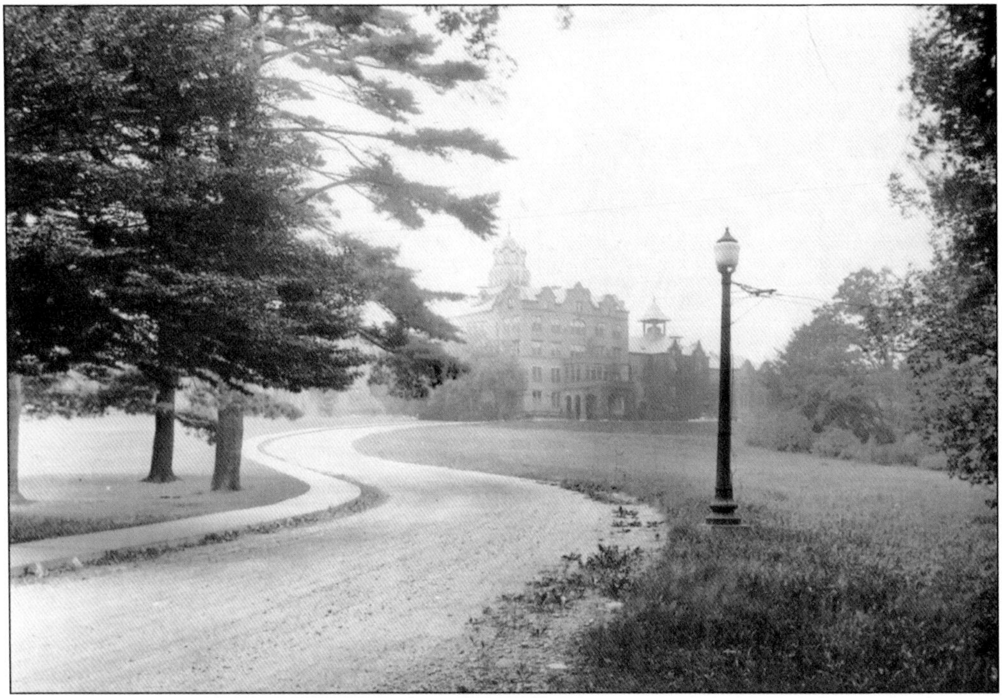

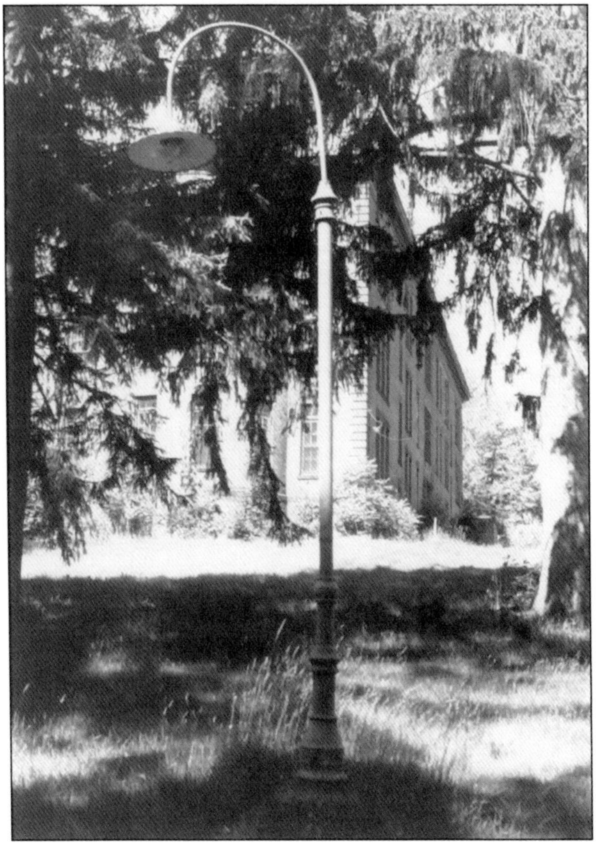

Streetlamps were installed in 1907 along the main entrance road to the hospital. In his request for a special state appropriation for this purpose, Supt. John Houston wrote, "Both foot path and driveway are long and circuitous, and at night the way is puzzling to those unacquainted with it, and gloomy, especially to the female employees." This atmospheric view confirms his opinion. Cast-iron "bishop's crook" streetlamps were also erected along the footpath from the main entrance to the central buildings.

Two

Inertia

Over the first 50 years of the 20th century, state hospitals grew very large as they were used for the care of an increasingly diverse population of people in need. They were asked to play a central role in response to many social ills and claimed a significant part of state budgets around the land. Northampton State Hospital admitted as many people with age-related senility as for all other diagnoses combined in 1948. By 1955, it housed 2,500 patients.

Acutely mentally ill patients were mixed with the chronically ill and the medically needy in old buildings bursting at their seams. The requirements of simply feeding and clothing and boarding such numbers of people taxed the staff to its limits. While patients continued to participate in industrial and occupational therapies, the presumption that the hospital served as a therapeutic environment was hard to maintain. Several medical treatments were adopted in the middle decades. Without a clear understanding of how these treatments worked, but with some encouraging results to urge them on, the doctors at Northampton, as at other state hospitals, administered Metrazol to induce a seizure and insulin to cause a coma. Later, electric shock replaced Metrazol and was widely used to treat people with many diagnoses.

Northampton State Hospital at its largest bore very little resemblance to the ideal vision of its founders. The overworked and underpaid staff scrambled to make do and worked to keep the peace on the wards. Their charges mostly sat, or sometimes stood because of the lack of chairs, or maybe paced in circles, as they endured the hopelessness and inertia of institutional life.

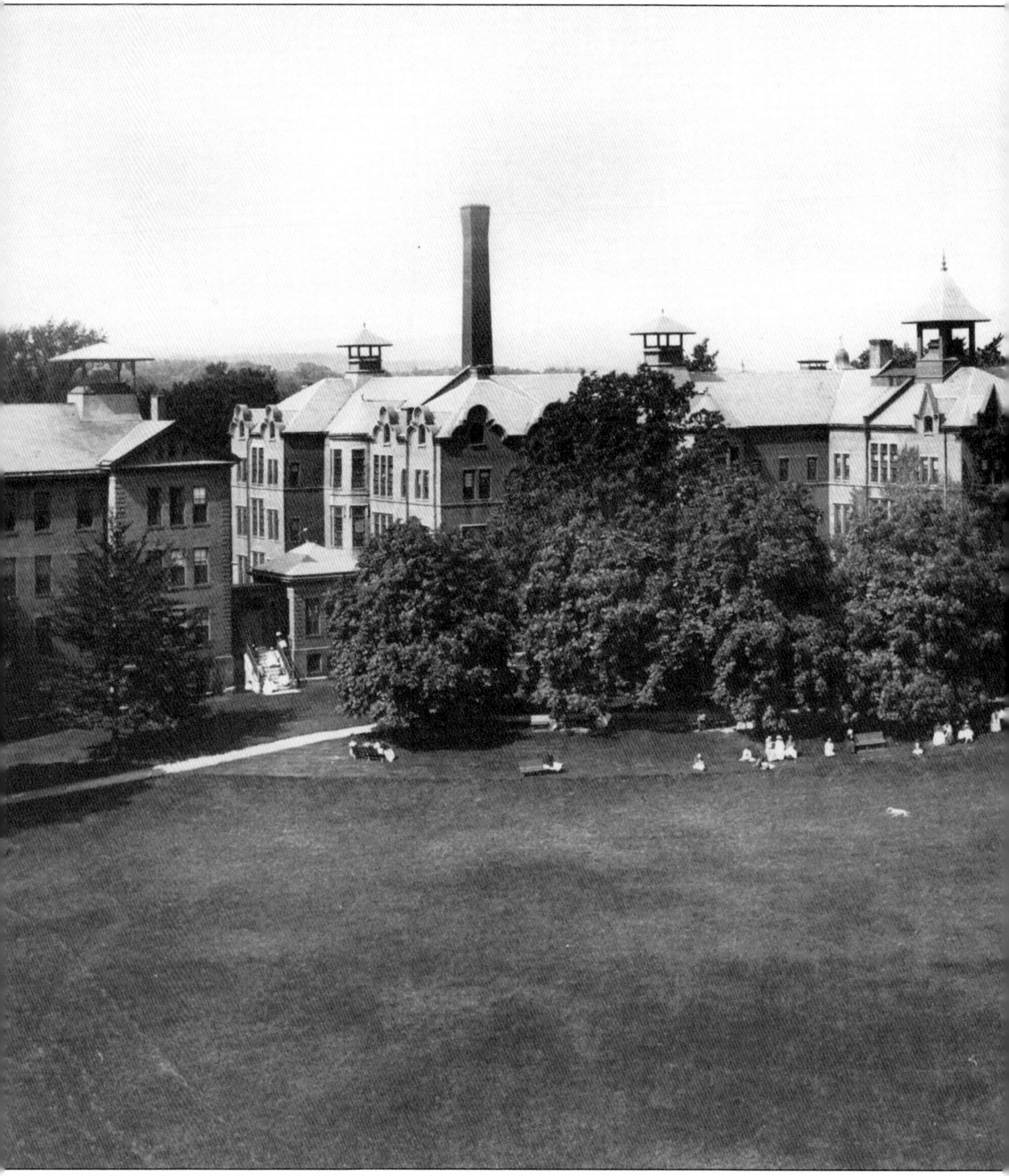

This shows the hospital at the height of its physical impressiveness in 1909, with the pleasure grounds surrounding the main building meticulously mowed and gently sloping, the driveway looking immaculate, and the trees majestic. A row of figures is seated along the edge of the meadow, facing the camera, which was placed on a temporary tower built especially so that this

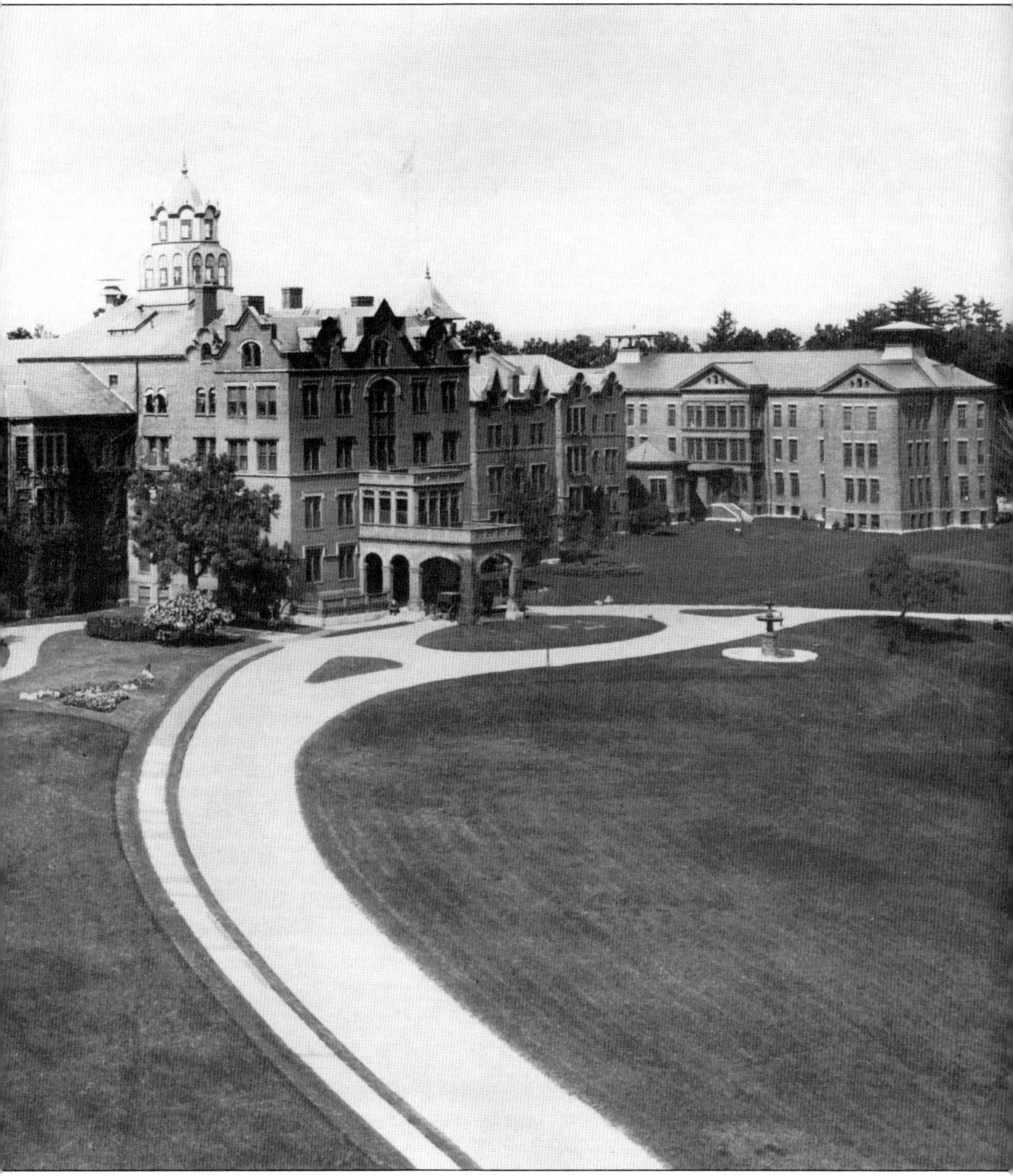

picture could be taken. No other image exists from this angle. Looking closely, one can make out a horse carriage in the covered entryway. Perhaps, it is picking up a patient or dropping off a visitor.

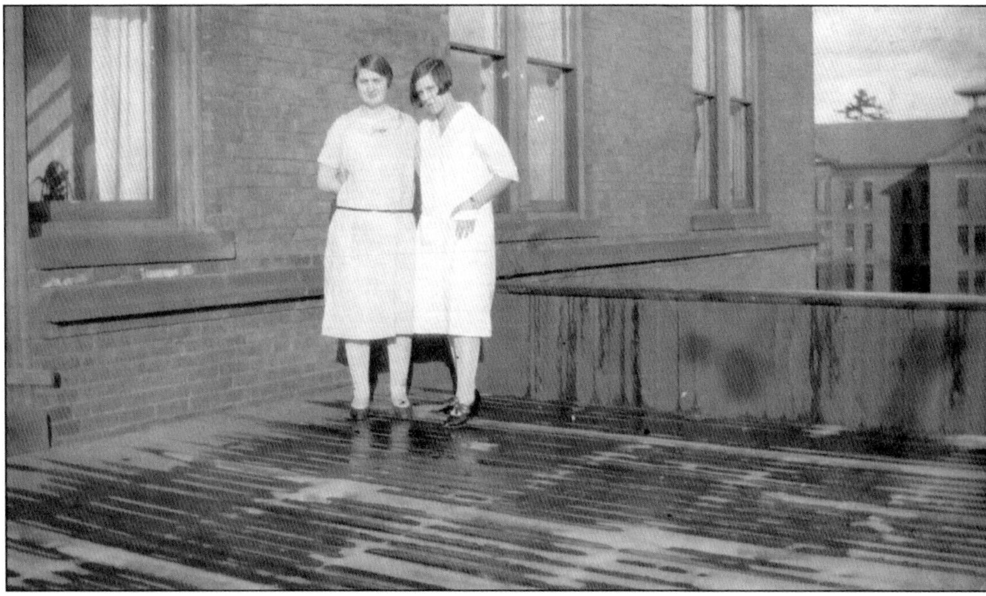

Pictured above in the 1920s, two women pose in the sun on the porch above the front entrance of the old main building. This is the only surviving photograph taken on the porch above the main entrance. Below is an man in his best clothes with the hospital as backdrop. Though they remain unidentified, they were part of the immense number of people whose lives were touched by the hospital in one way or another. Overall, Northampton State Hospital admitted nearly 65,000 patients over the course of its history. Very few photographs survive of the patients, even though they dramatically outnumbered the staff. The selection of photographs that survives is mostly centered around the employees, who had the means and ability to record and capture their days on film.

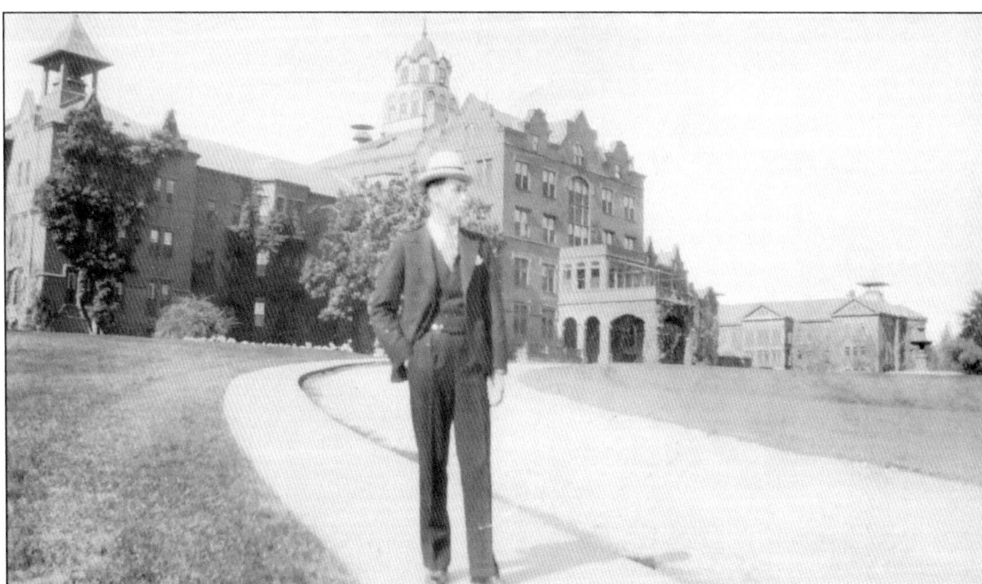

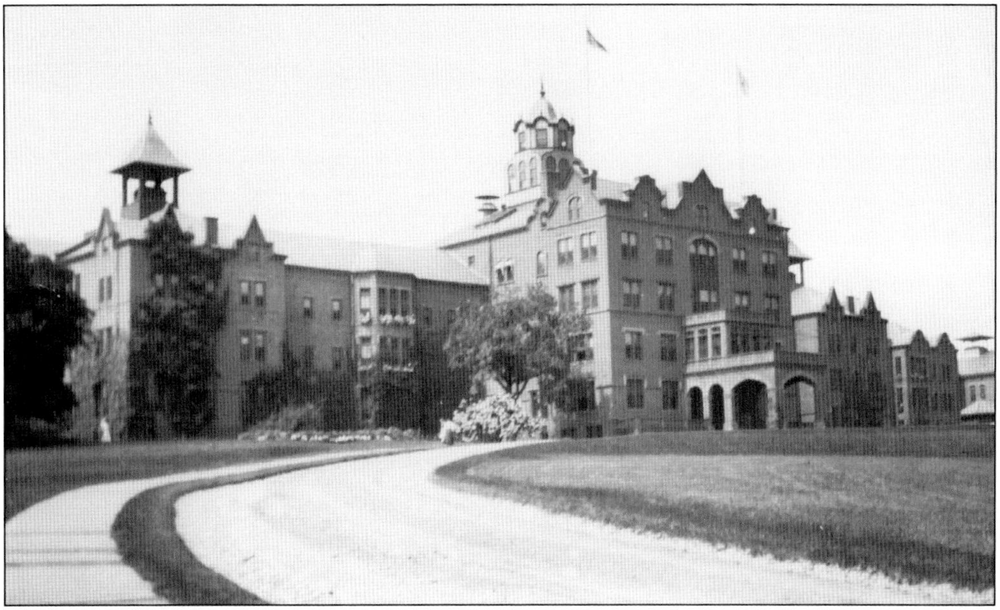

This photograph from around 1905 shows the remodeled ventilation towers. "A complete system of forced ventilation in connection with the heating is indispensable to give purity to the air of a hospital for the insane" was a unanimous resolution by the Association of Medical Superintendents. In later years, these ventilation towers were mistakenly seen as guard towers, which fit into the reputation of the hospital as a prison-like institution.

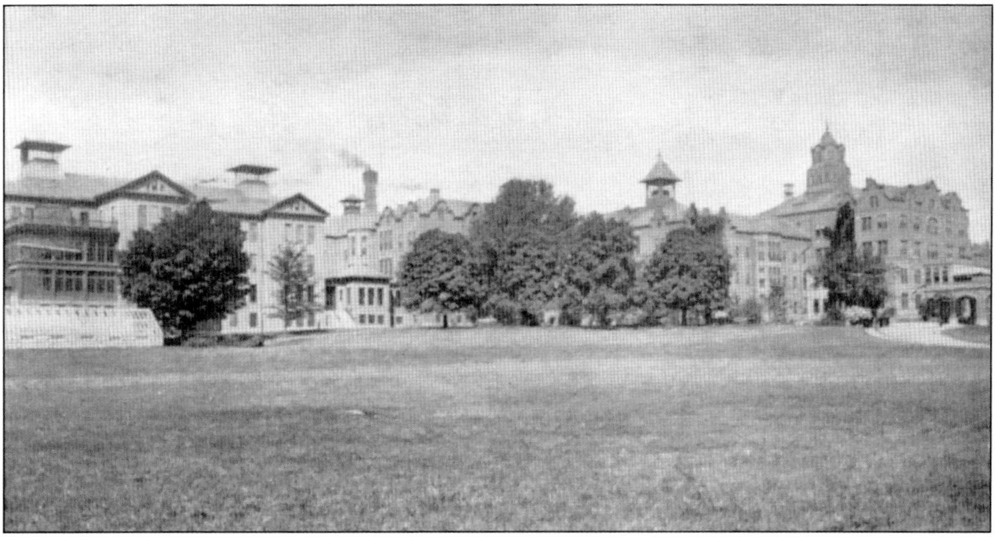

This found postcard, dated sometime around 1905, says, "Hoping you are having a pleasant time, from Emil." One might try to imagine the sender of such a card. Was he a patient? Was he a family member of a patient, or a friend, or perhaps an employee? Who would write such a card and send it? It is unknown how many postcards were printed of the hospital over the years, but several designs existed and can still be found in thrift stores and postcard collections, near and far.

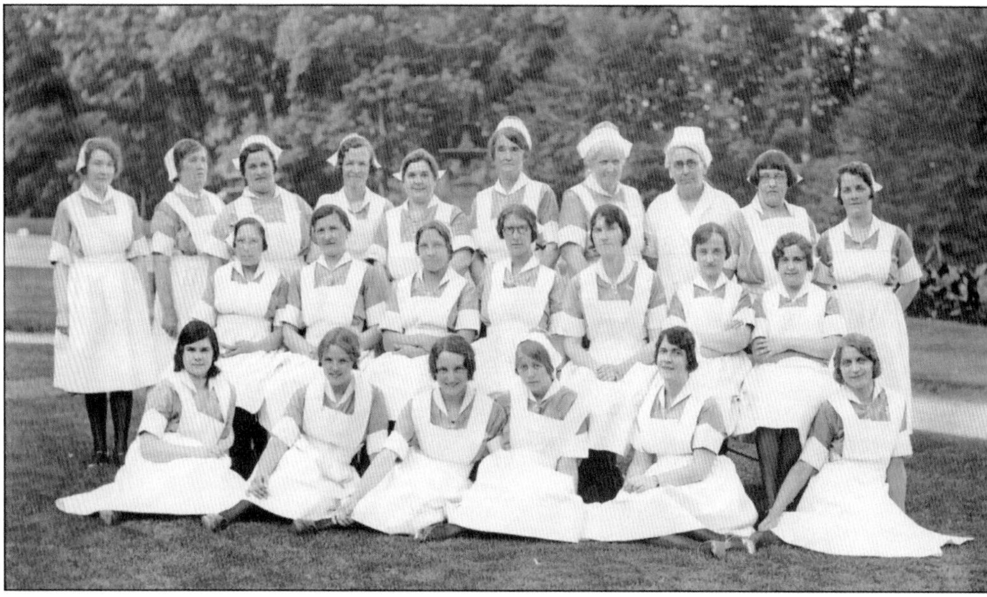

"The supervisors are not graduate nurses but are hardworking, kind, experienced men, who saw that the patients were clean, clothed, and comfortably cared for under a moderately rigid sort of discipline," reported a state inspector. In the mid-20th century, custodial care trumped any form of treatment. The attendants kept the system operating under trying conditions. Experience was their guide. Patient abuse often went unobserved or unreported. Acts of kindness and generosity would go untold. A shortage of attendants was a constant concern. In a typical year in the first half of the 20th century, between 60 and 70 percent of attendants had been in the job less than a year. It was not unusual to have 40 percent of the funded attendant positions unfilled. While mechanics and craftsmen worked 8-hour days beginning in 1906, attendants still worked 10 hours a day in 1930.

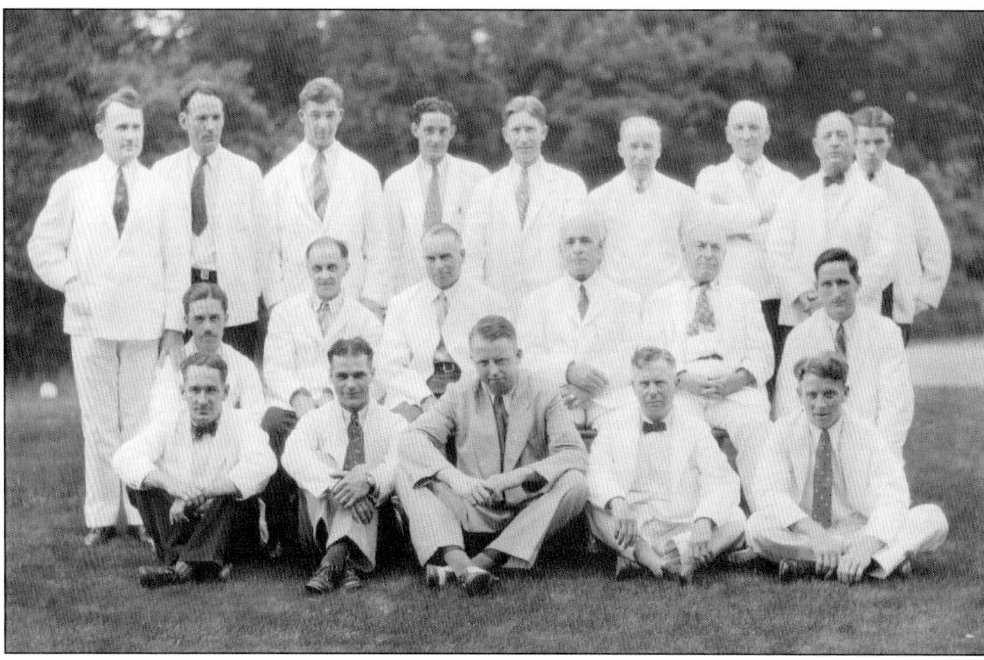

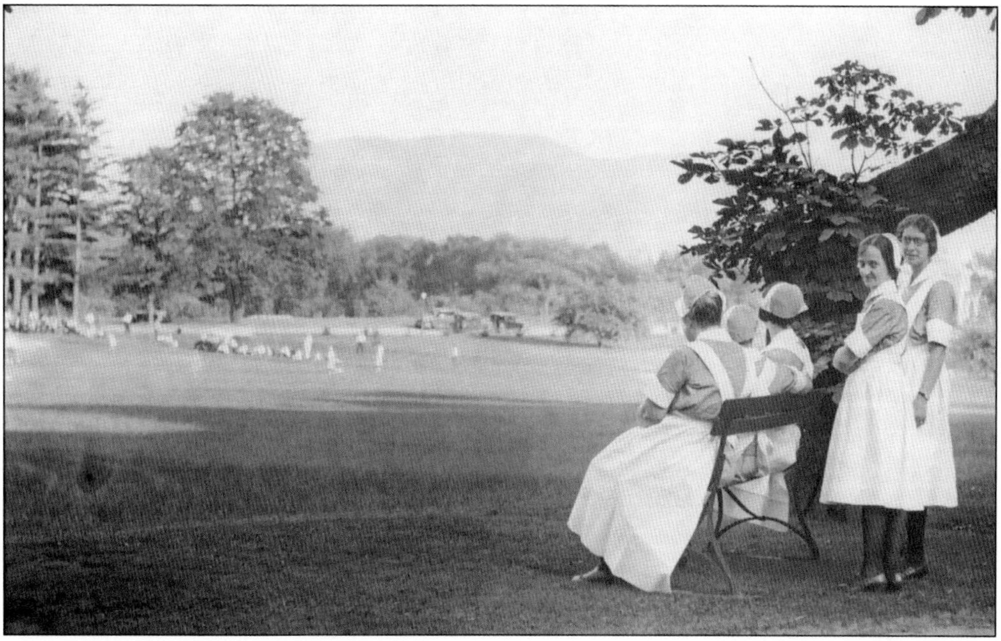

The psychiatric ideal in the 19th century, as expressed by Thomas Kirkbride, suggested that "the views should exhibit life in its active forms, stirring objects at a little distance are desirable." In this rare outdoor scene, the grand scale of the front lawn of the hospital can be glimpsed, featuring five attendants in the foreground, a game of baseball, the driveway in the middle distance, and the Holyoke Range in the far distance. The hospital was hailed for its beautiful setting and its exquisite views, which had originally been chosen to provide a context of natural beauty, hope, and serenity for the patients. The beautiful grounds remained a treasured asset of the institution until it closed.

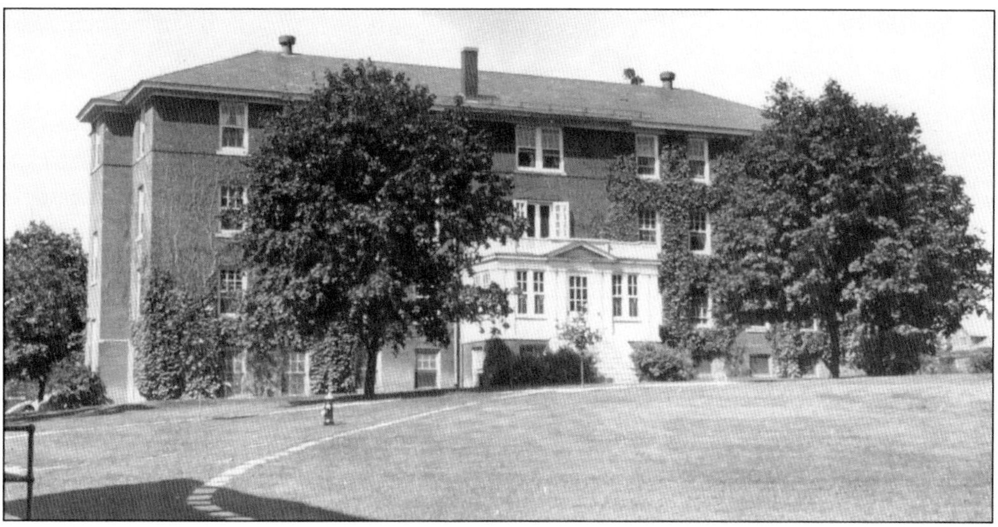

The South Attendants' Home, shown here, and its twin North Attendants' Home opened in 1920. Female workers lived at the south, while male workers initially resided at the north, which was converted to a married couples' home in the 1930s. Speaking of her experience living here in 1935, an employee said, "About five o'clock in the morning you could hear the patients that were already rising from bed. I could make out who they were, too, from my ward."

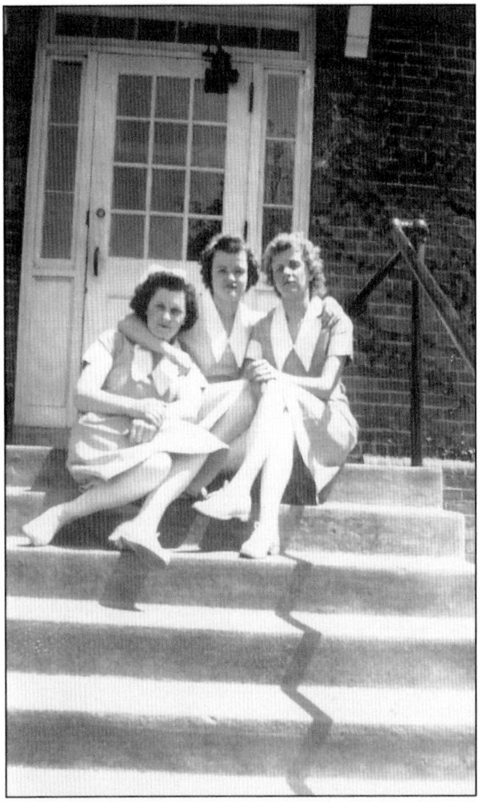

Posing on the side steps of the South Attendants' Home are employees Alice Baceski, Gert Zagrodnik, and Virginia Kielbowicz. Long work hours and communal living made for deep and lasting friendships. Zagrodnik is captured in a moment of repose in the occupational therapy room in the image below.

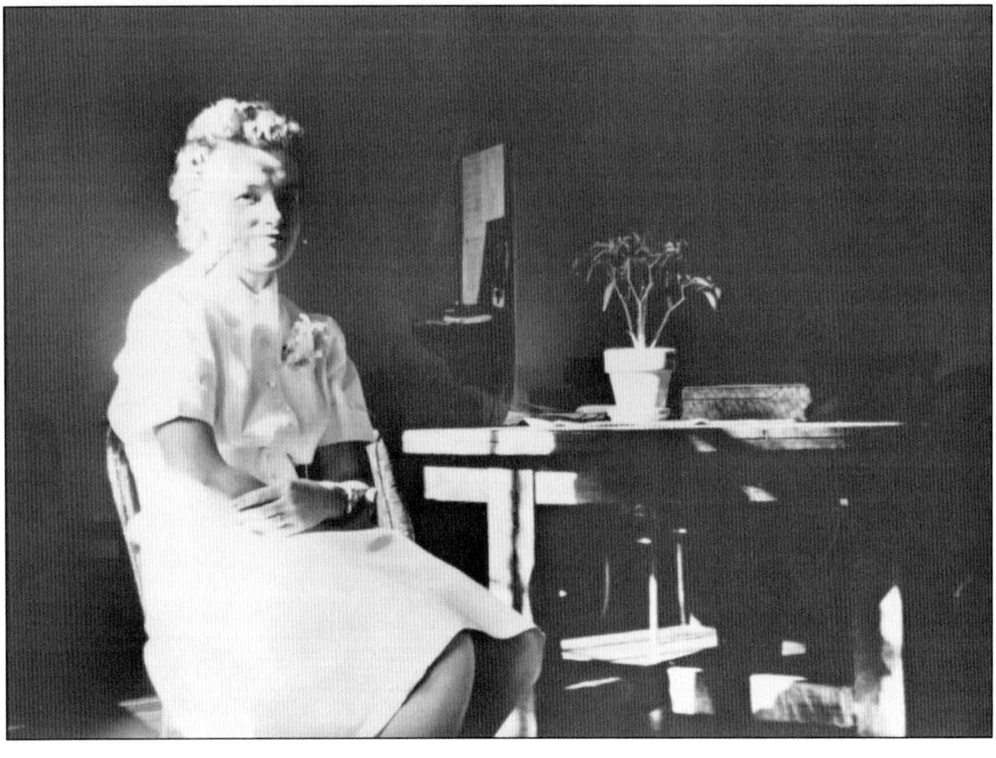

Few workers at the hospital owned cars in the 1930s. A female attendant reported, "Once in a while a guy would have a car, and we would all get in and we'd overcrowd it, and off we'd go to some dance in Holyoke." This 1930 roadster belonged to Dominic Mazilli, shown in his white attendant's uniform with the corner of the Nurses' Home in the background.

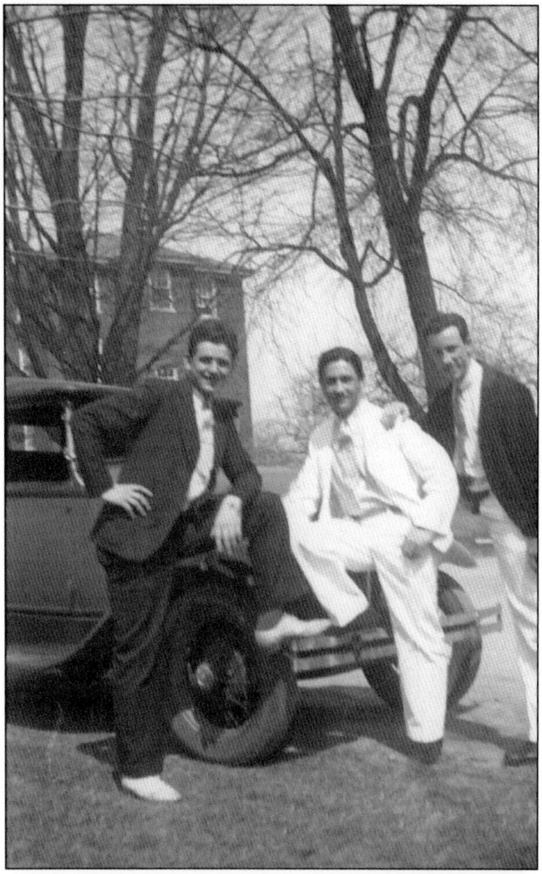

Good and plentiful food was one of the benefits of working at the hospital. Much of the food was grown or raised on the grounds, with all the cooking and baking done on the premises. Food and housing helped induce people to take work at the hospital for relatively low wages and long hours. This is the employee cafeteria in 1930.

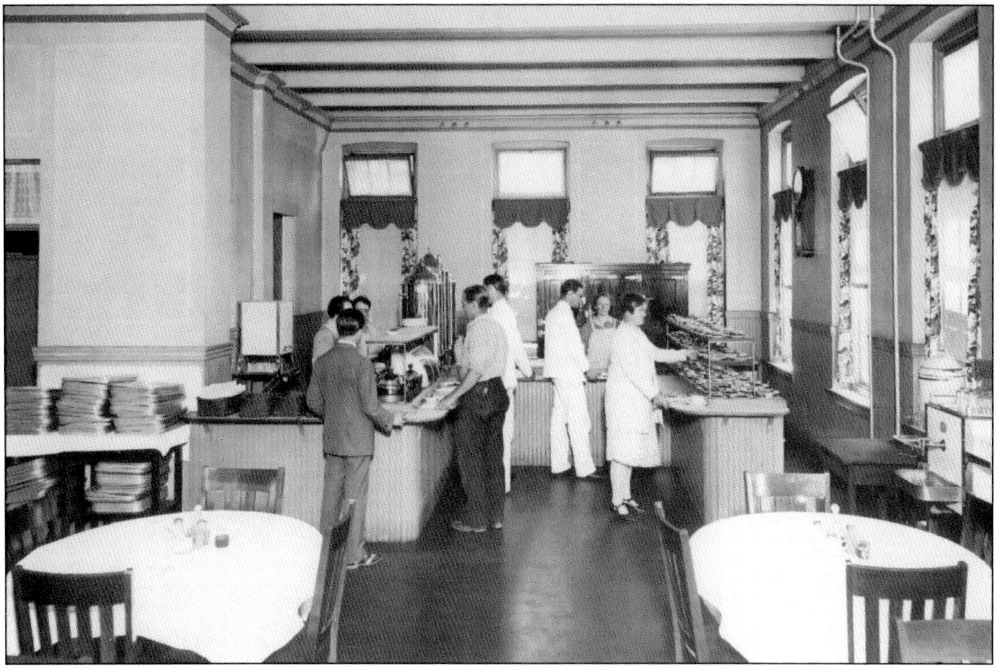

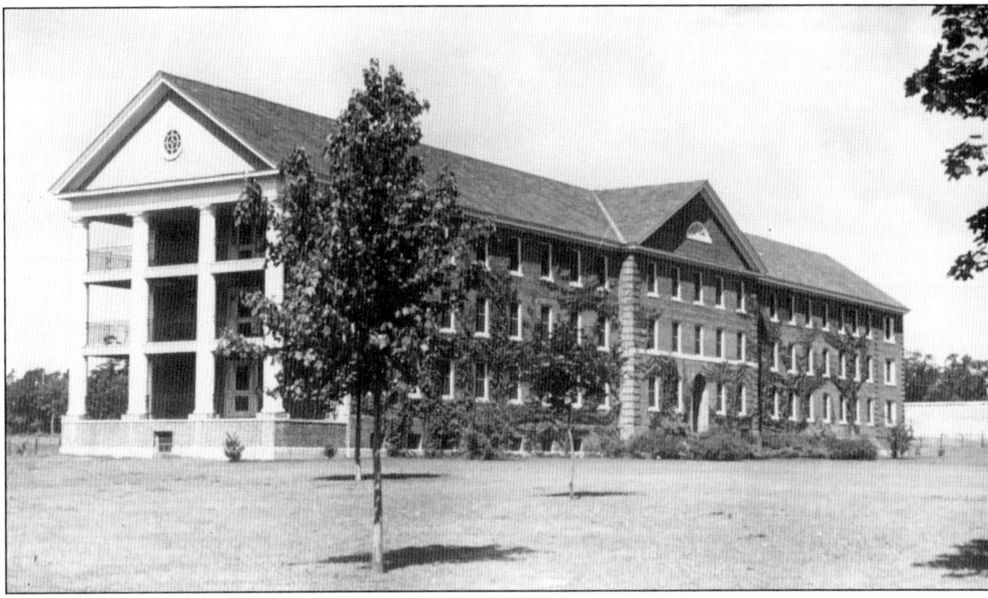

The last major residential building to be constructed, the Male Attendants' Home opened in 1933. There were 100 single rooms and a smoking and card room in the basement. Below, ward attendants await the change of shift in the spring of 1936. In 1990, there were plans to reuse the empty building for administrative and clinical offices as part of a new, renovated hospital. At that time, it was renamed in honor of Dr. Shirley M. Gallup. Today, it is being considered for redevelopment as a hotel.

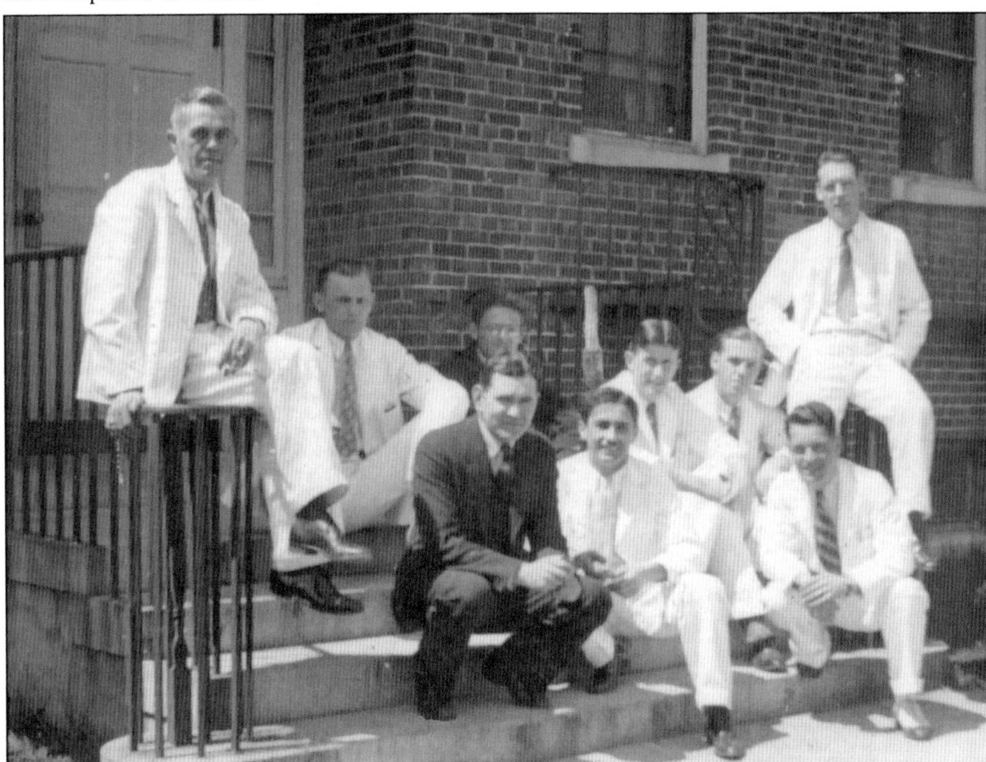

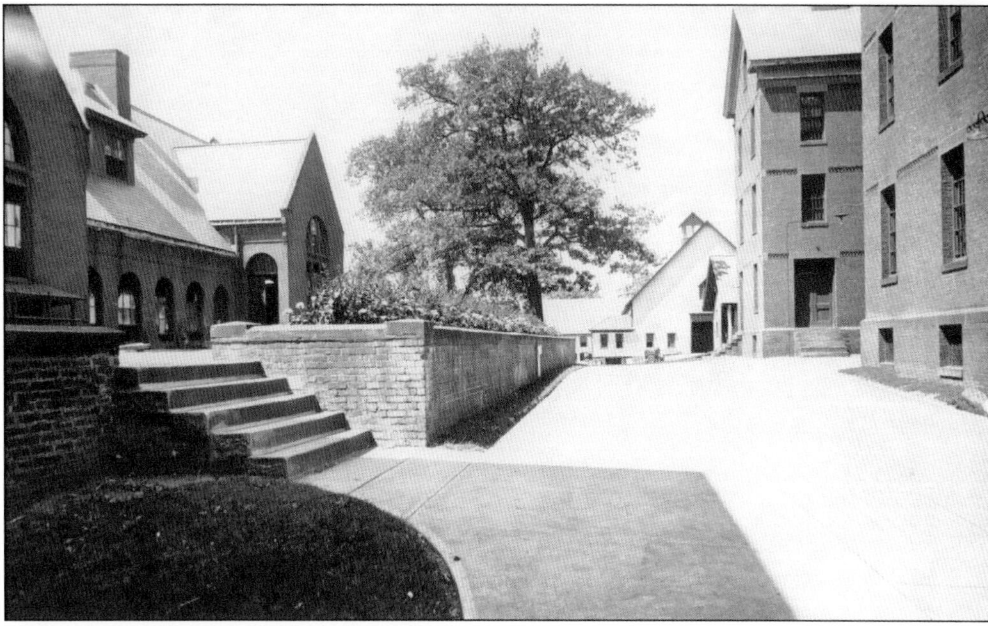

This unusual view shows the rear of the main buildings, looking out toward the barn. On the right is the 1884 building that was converted to a dormitory for patients working on the farm, and it was used in that capacity until 1934. On the left is a complex of buildings housing the carpentry, machine, and paint shops and the old power plant. This was all demolished to build the Olander Cafeteria in 1936.

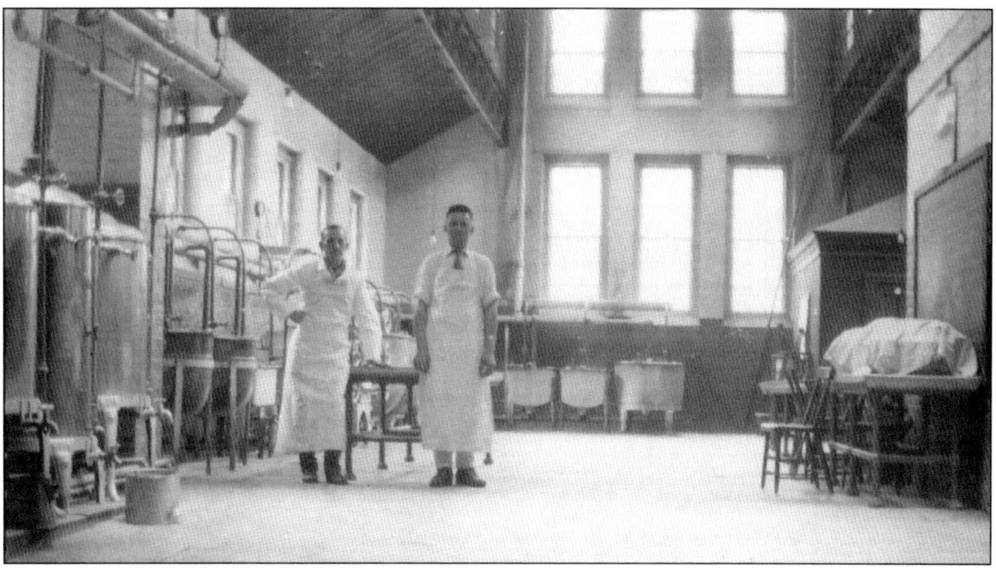

Two employees stand in the kitchen before the renovations of the mid-1930s. There were always patients staffing the kitchens as well. A former patient writes, "I had a job in the kitchen, I was a dishwasher and mopped floors. We, the Kitchen People, would play cards at a little table downstairs. I think there I didn't feel so much like a State Hospital Patient. I think it was the Apron. I always thought the food was good. One thing that Northampton had I really liked was the tart pies, the damn things were enough to drive me out of my head, or belly, because I couldn't get enough of them."

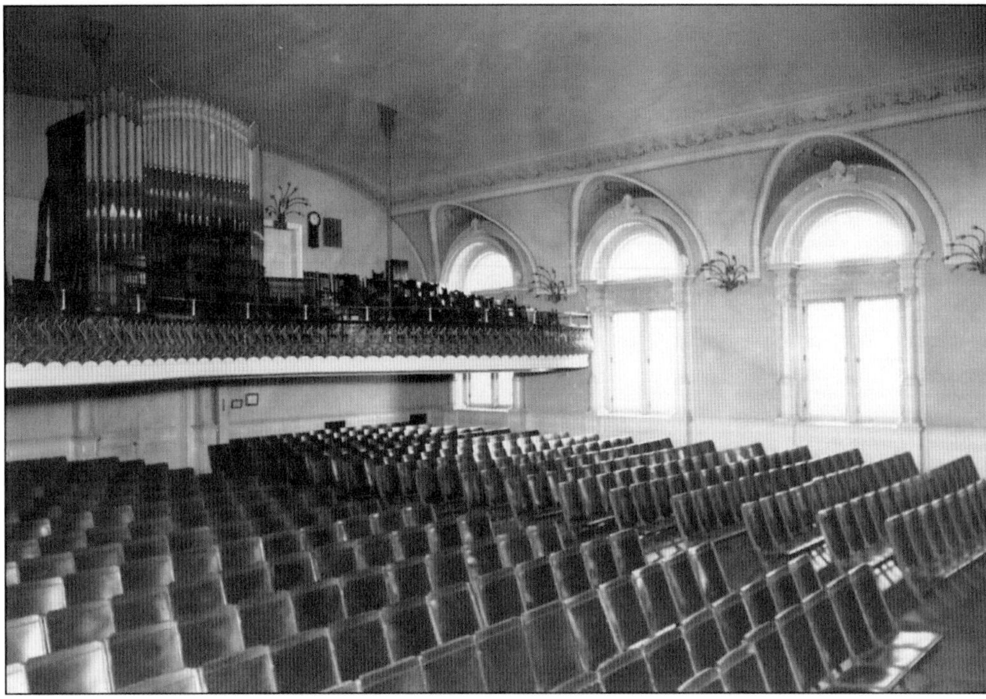

The hospital chapel dates to 1895 when the central section of the main buildings was renovated. It included a gallery at one end and a large stage at the other and had a capacity of 600. The interior was finished in white and gold in Norman style. The retiring superintendent, Dr. Edward Nims, as a memorial to his late wife, installed the pipe organ in 1897. The chapel was the center for many social events. In the photograph below, the chapel has been decorated for Halloween by patients, with the help of occupational therapy staff.

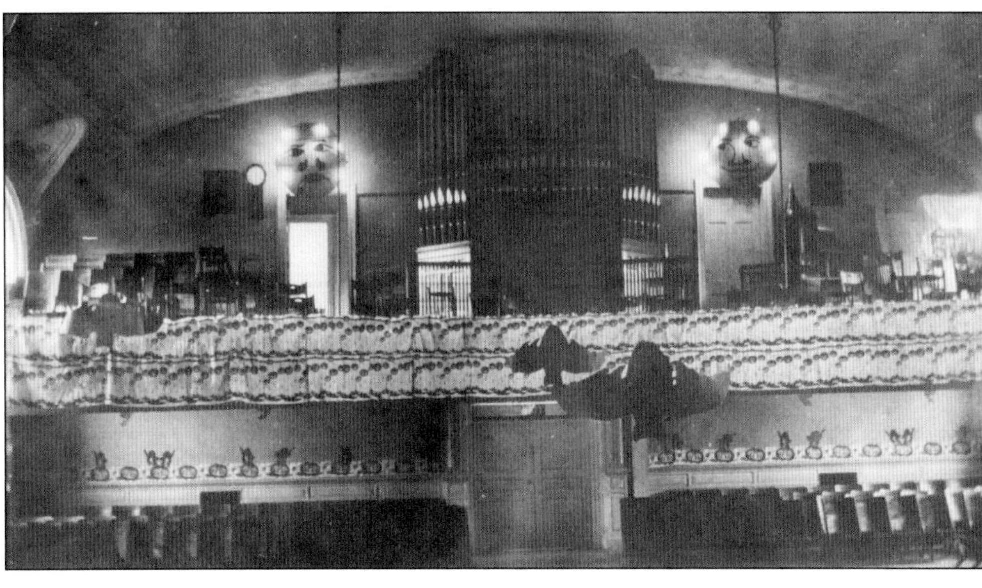

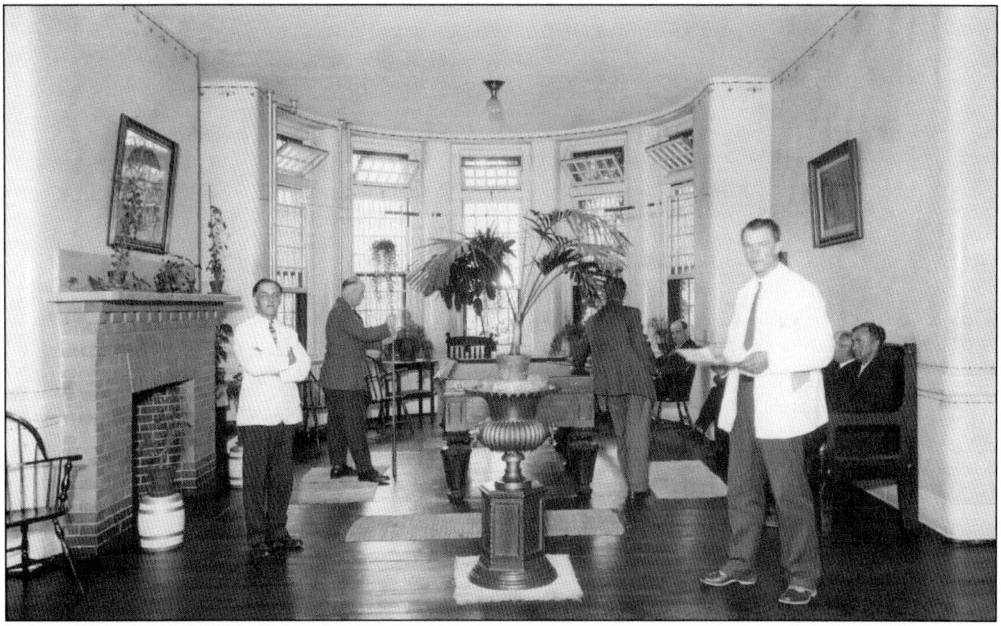

Patients and staff pose in the dayroom on the first floor of the male wards near the central entrance, called Lower North 1. Just beyond this room are the rotunda and the front door of the hospital. Male patients who had few behavioral problems lived here. They could leave the ward during the day, and most worked, in some capacity, in one of the departments. Dr. B. Edwin Zawacki, the chief of the male service, stands on the right in this 1930 view.

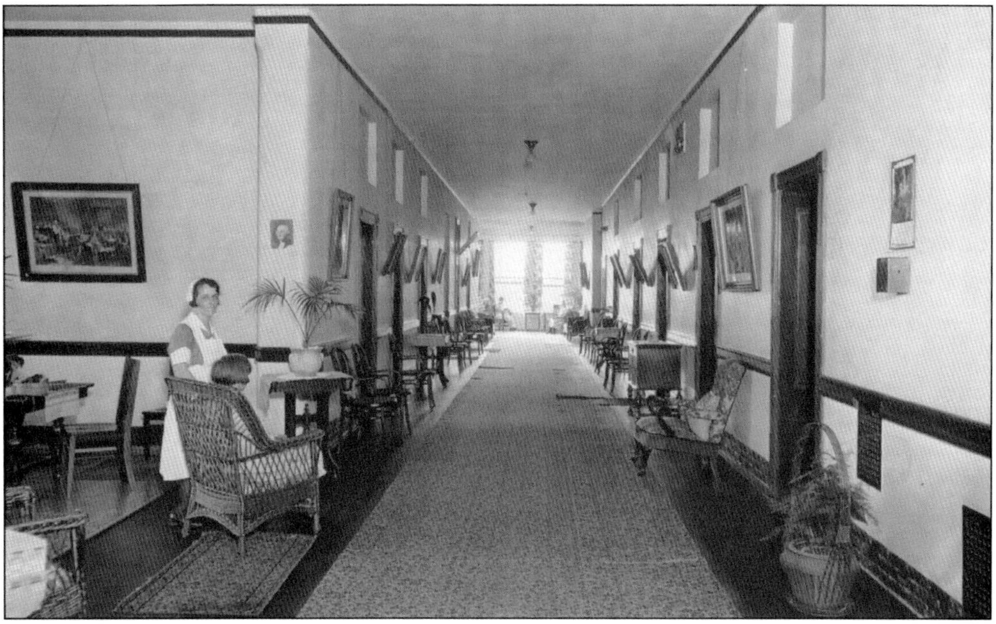

This is the corresponding female ward on the south side of the central offices, called Lower South 1. More than any other ward, this maintained the quality and feeling of the building when new, including the furnishings of an inviting domestic interior. Even when the single rooms were crowded with two patients, the quality of life on this ward was relatively good. This view is also from 1930.

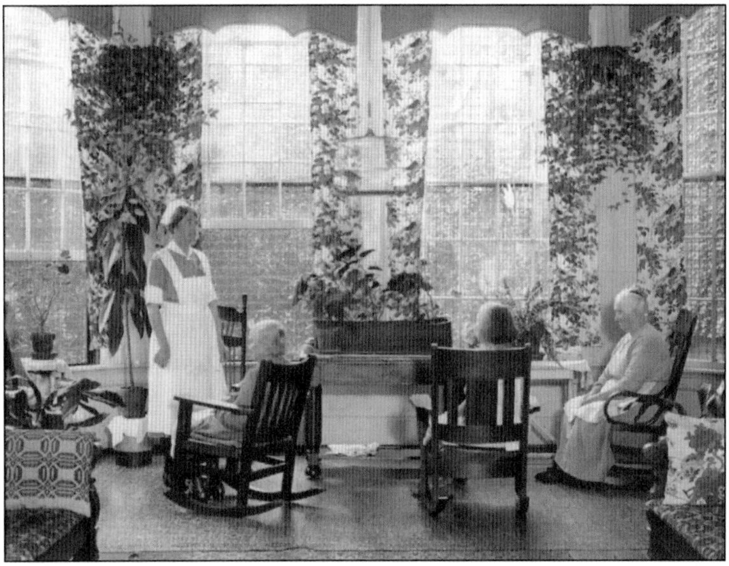

This eight-sided bay with large windows was built in 1915 at the end of the corridor of Lower South 1 and was said in an annual report to "make the life of the patients much pleasanter, affording more sunshine and cheer to the wards which they adjoin." This first-floor ward was the showplace of the hospital. A Mrs. Bickford, the nurse in charge, poses with three patients.

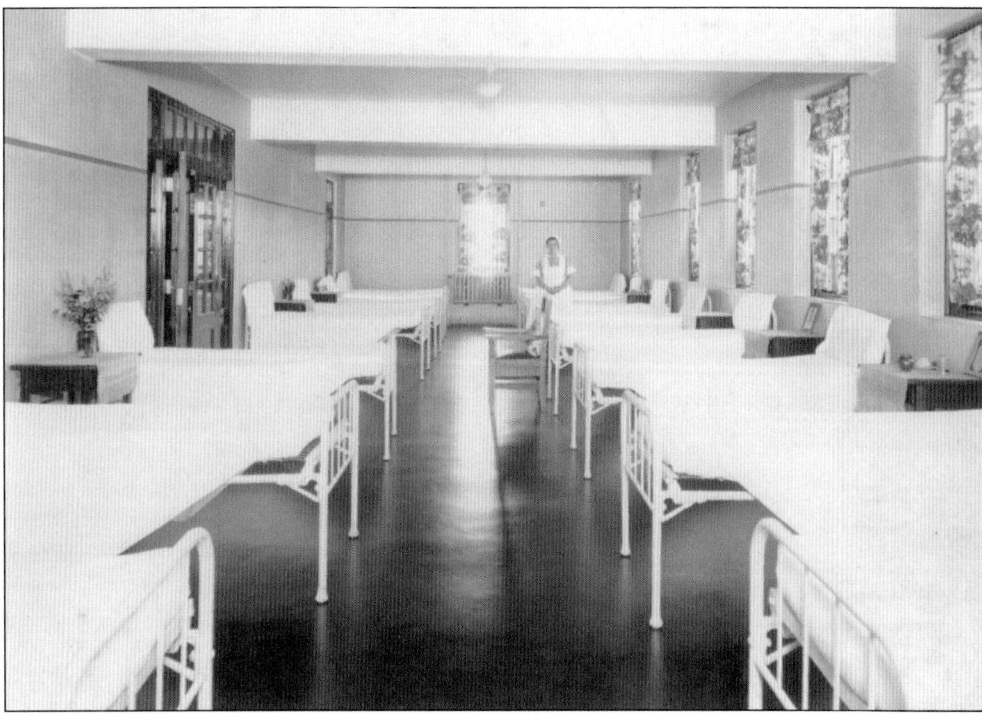

As neat as this ward appears, it was not the intended sleeping arrangement for patients in the original design. "The great majority of patients would strenuously object to such an arrangement," wrote Thomas Kirkbride. This photograph marks the transition of the hospital wards from full occupancy toward overcrowding. By 1945, most of the wards were so crowded that the beds were touching, with little or no space to move around comfortably. Privacy is a collective value and a human right, which is impossible to uphold in conditions of hospital overcrowding. It is the first and most basic personal right to be lost in such a setting.

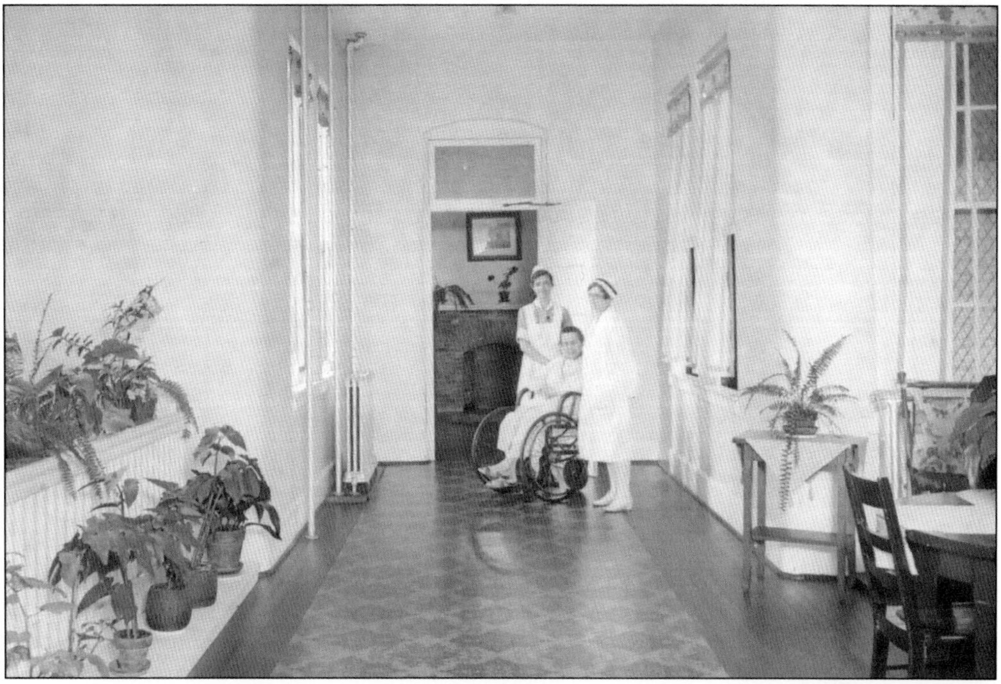

The infirmary buildings were in operation by 1905 and provided a focus for those with acute medical needs. Their wards filled with elderly, frail patients as their numbers increased in the hospital. It would be a rare sight to see nearly empty corridors.

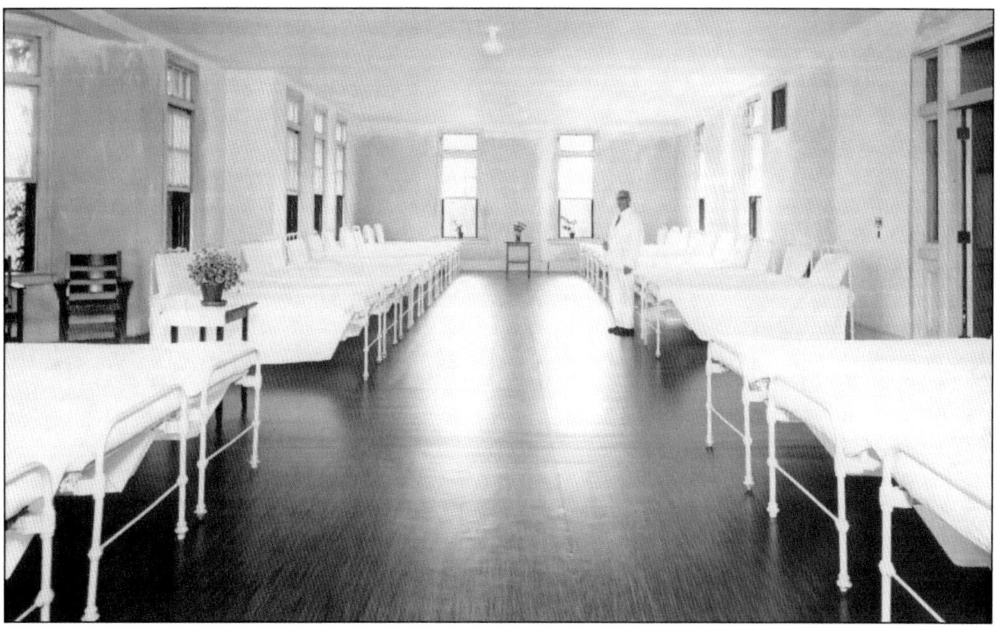

"Patients that are excitable rarely do well in large wards," cautioned Thomas Kirkbride in his design guide for hospitals. Here is a full dormitory for male patients with the beds almost touching. Originally, the wards were to house between 15 and 20 patients each. By 1900, the wards had grown, however, to serve many more patients than could comfortably sleep and move around. Overcrowding would not be alleviated until the late 1970s and 1980s.

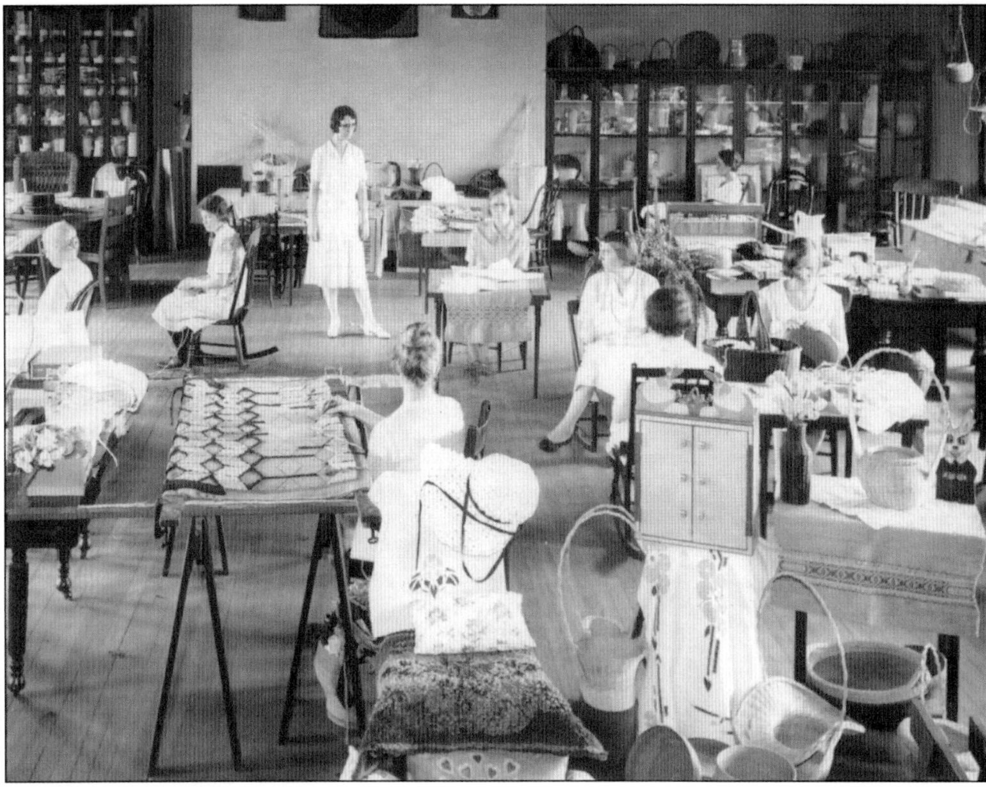

Occupational therapy was women's work in 1930 and for nearly 30 years after that. The large occupational therapy room in the back of the central building afforded space for knitting, sewing, quilting, hat making, basketry, and more. The person standing in the back is likely Vera Mathieu, head of occupational therapy.

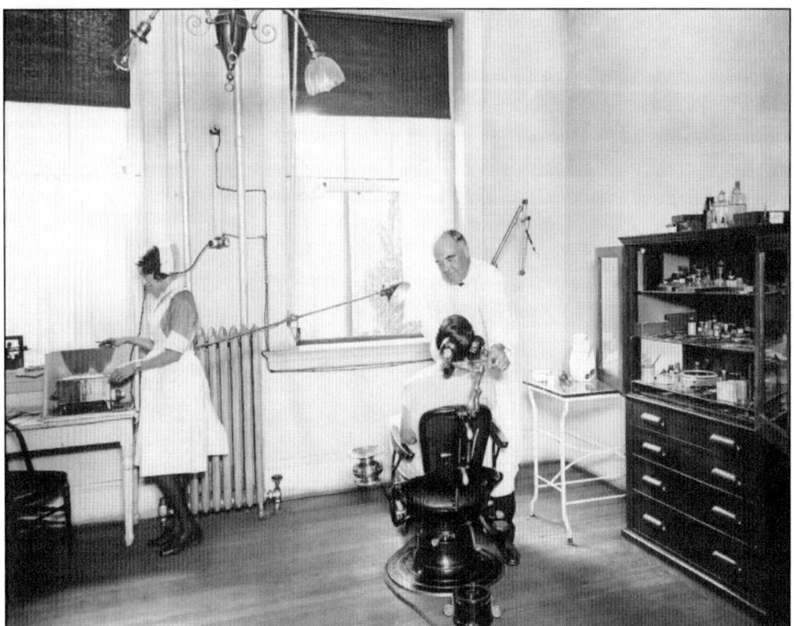

The teeth of all new patients were examined by the hospital's dentist, Dr. Lucien Harris, in this suite in the center of the main buildings. In the year 1934, he gave 4,315 treatments, which included fillings, plates, cleanings, and extractions. He retired in 1943.

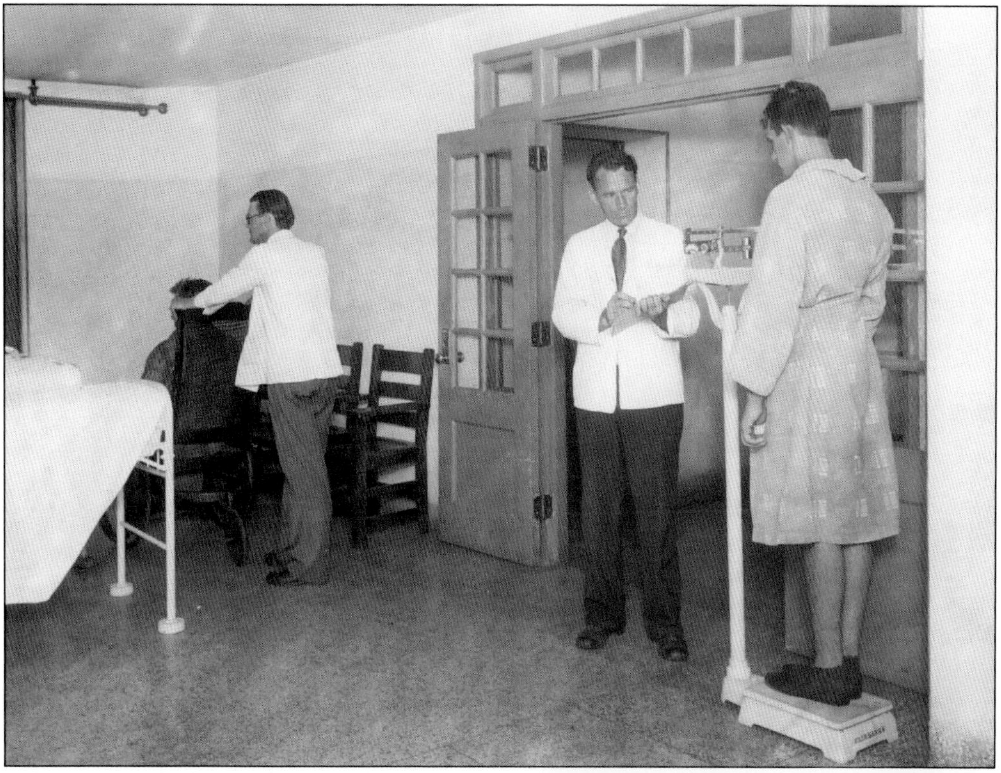

Admission to the hospital involved undergoing a physical and psychological examination, followed by enforced bed rest. Usually in the third week in residence, the case would be discussed "in abstract" by a conference led by the assistant superintendent "relative to diagnosis, treatment, and disposition," reported a state inspector in 1952. Should symptoms not improve, one had every chance of staying in the hospital long term. In that case, a psychiatric examination would be scheduled once a year but often did not occur due to staff shortages.

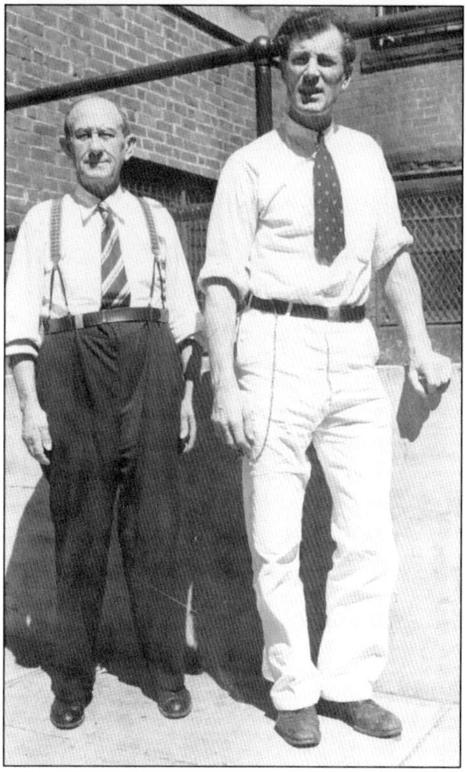

Foster Wheeler, on the right, was the hydrotherapist on the male side in the 1930s. He is shown here with a man believed to be his patient assistant. Many shops of the hospital had patient workers, who, because of their skill and their longevity in the "job," were sometimes mistaken for employees. A longtime worker in the bookbindery was several times mistaken for the boss by hospital staff visiting that shop.

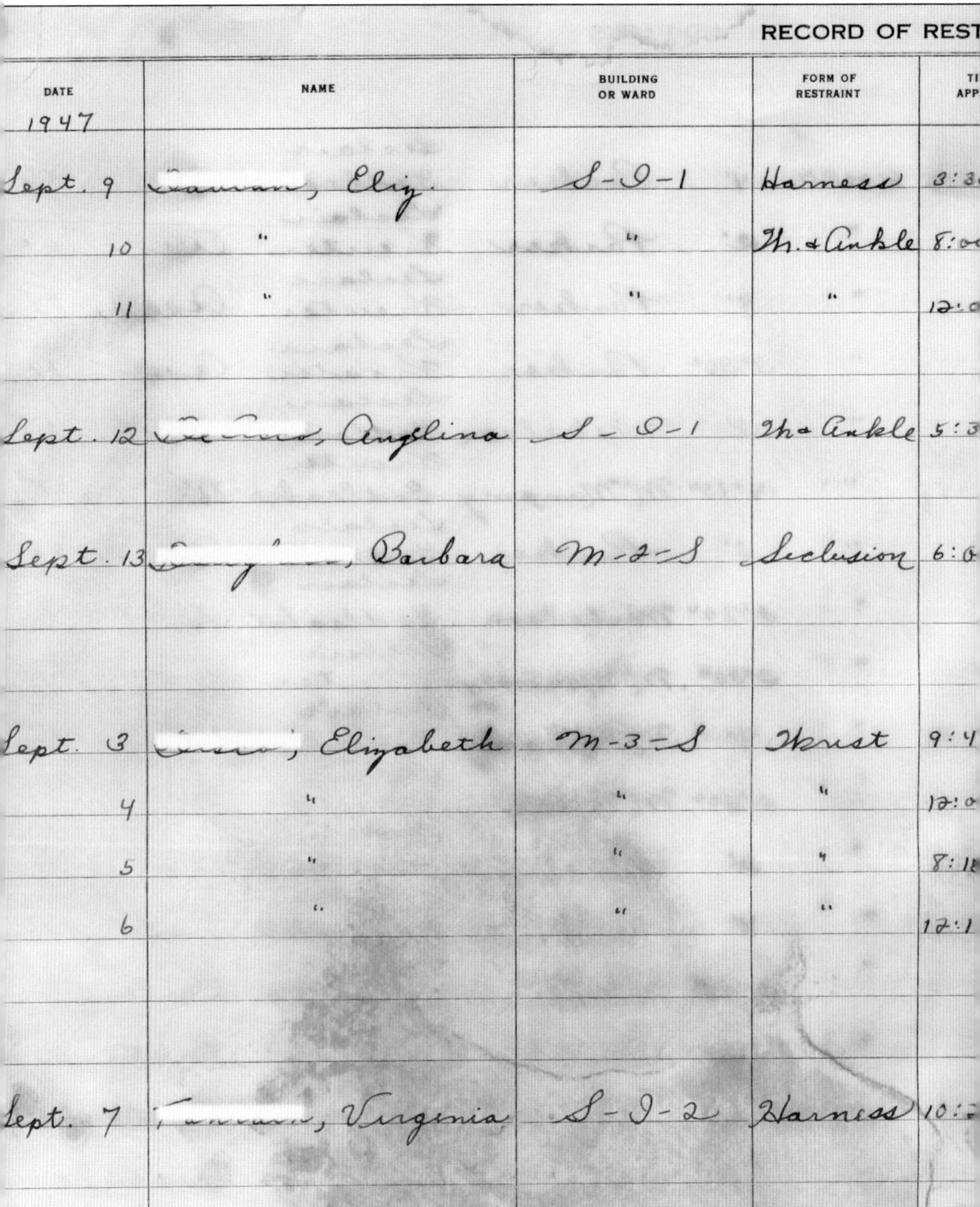

RECORD OF REST

DATE	NAME	BUILDING OR WARD	FORM OF RESTRAINT	TI APP
1947				
Sept. 9	[illegible], Eliz.	S-I-1	Harness	3:3
10	"	"	H. & Ankle	8:0
11	"	"	"	12:0
Sept. 12	[illegible], Anglina	S-I-1	H.& Ankle	5:3
Sept. 13	[illegible], Barbara	M-2-S	Seclusion	6:0
Sept. 3	[illegible], Elizabeth	M-3-S	Wrist	9:4
4	"	"	"	12:0
5	"	"	"	8:1
6	"	"	"	12:1
Sept. 7	[illegible], Virginia	S-I-2	Harness	10:

Even in times of overcrowding and understaffing, records were kept meticulously, perhaps as a tool for ordering what could not be ordered otherwise. This 1947 sheet records, among other entries, a 16-hour, continuous restraint of a female patient. At the same time, long-term "quiet," or chronic, patients received little attention, as employees at Northampton State Hospital

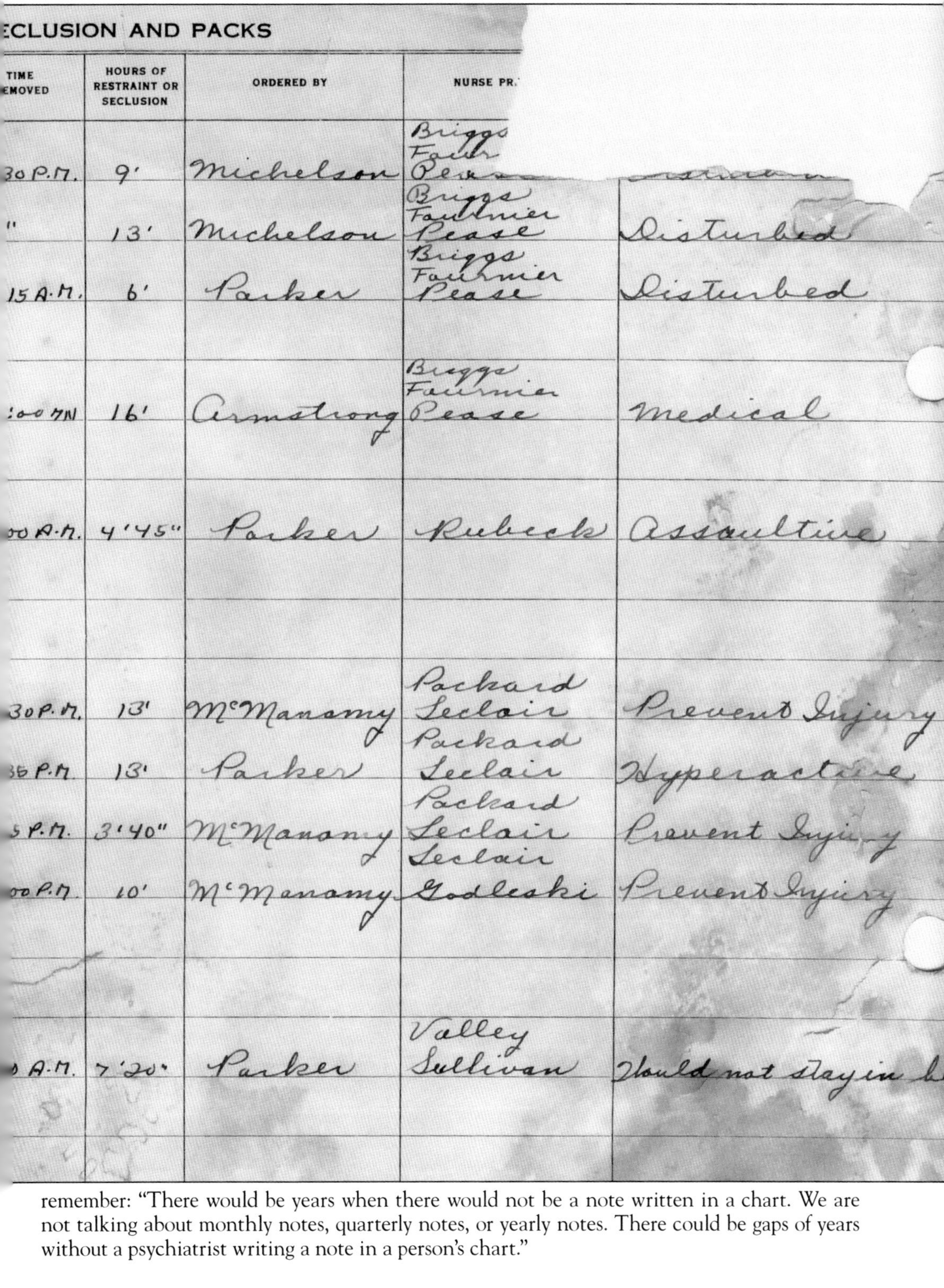

ECLUSION AND PACKS

TIME REMOVED	HOURS OF RESTRAINT OR SECLUSION	ORDERED BY	NURSE PR.	
30 P.M.	9'	Michelson	Briggs Four Pease	
"	13'	Michelson	Briggs Faulmier Pease	Disturbed
15 A.M.	6'	Parker	Briggs Faurmier Pease	Disturbed
:00 PM	16'	Armstrong	Briggs Faurmier Pease	Medical
00 A.M.	4'45"	Parker	Rubeck	Assaultive
30 P.M.	13'	McManamy	Packard Seclair	Prevent Injury
35 P.M.	13'	Parker	Packard Seclair	Hyperactive
5 P.M.	3'40"	McManamy	Packard Seclair	Prevent Injury
00 P.M.	10'	McManamy	Seclair Godleski	Prevent Injury
A.M.	7'20"	Parker	Valley Sullivan	Would not stay in b

remember: "There would be years when there would not be a note written in a chart. We are not talking about monthly notes, quarterly notes, or yearly notes. There could be gaps of years without a psychiatrist writing a note in a person's chart."

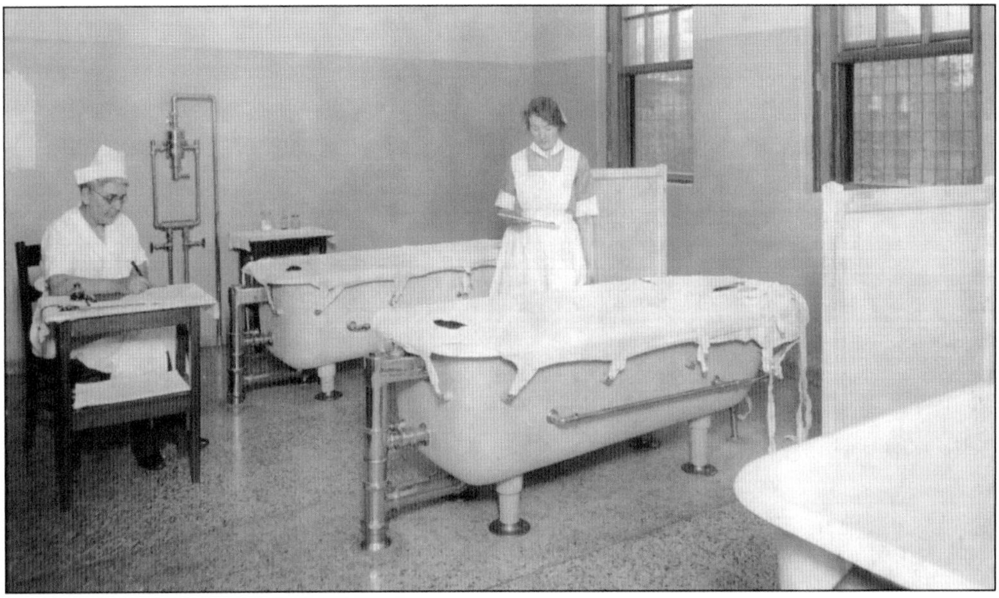

Hydrotherapy was a widely used treatment for calming manic or overexcited patients before the advent of psychotropic drugs and was practiced at the hospital since at least 1898. The hydrotherapy suites were located in the basement of the fourth wards on each side of the main building. One type of hydrotherapy involved securing patients in these large tubs with warm flowing water. Another hydrotherapy treatment involved immobilizing and cooling agitated patients by tightly wrapping them, first with a wet cotton blanket and then by several chilled blankets. "Wet packs" could be lifesaving for patients who were wildly overstimulated. Unfortunately, around 1950, state inspectors found that a patient might be put in restraints or packs "at the slightest indication that he or she may be getting excited, irritable, overacting, or threatening." Hydrotherapy was discontinued in 1953.

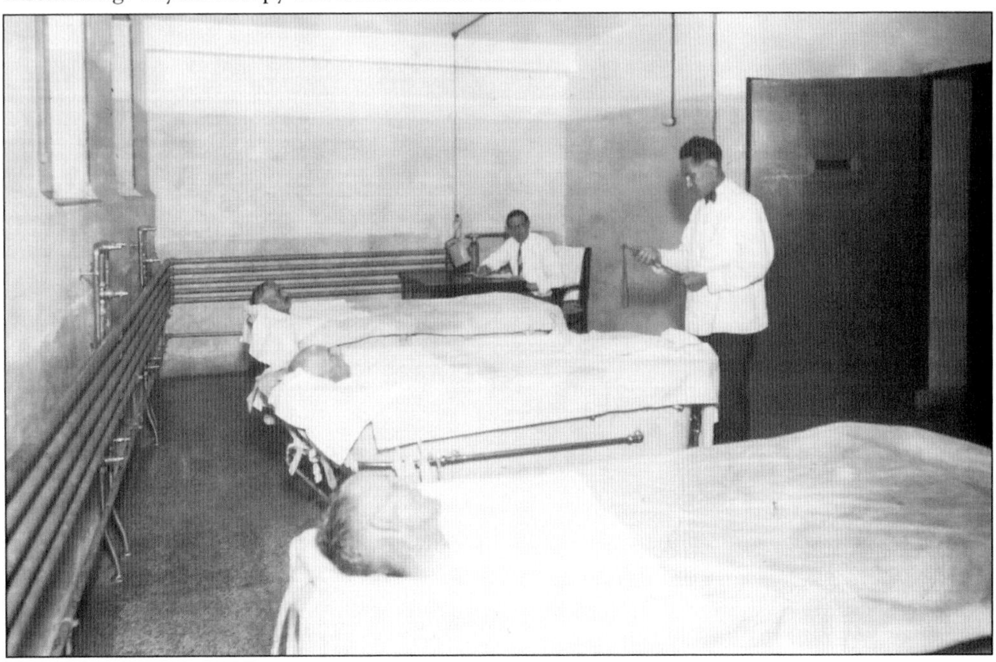

"In the highest part of the structure, as in a dome, the water tanks should be provided for." A daily consumption of 10,000 gallons of hot and cold water was estimated for baths, treatments, and water closets in every part of the building, with "tanks to contain more than this amount placed in the dome," advised Thomas Kirkbride. The dome also contained an observatory, "from which the most magnificent prospect in the Connecticut Valley can be obtained," marveled the first trustees of the hospital.

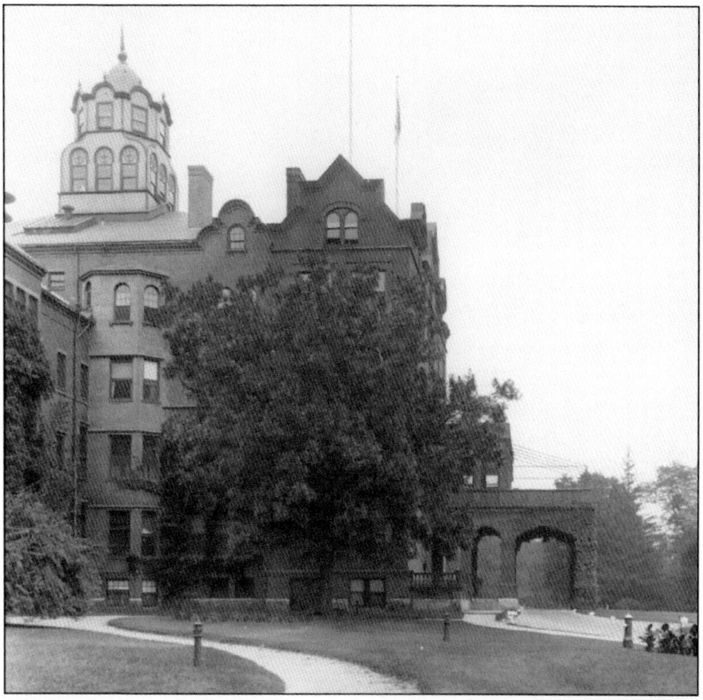

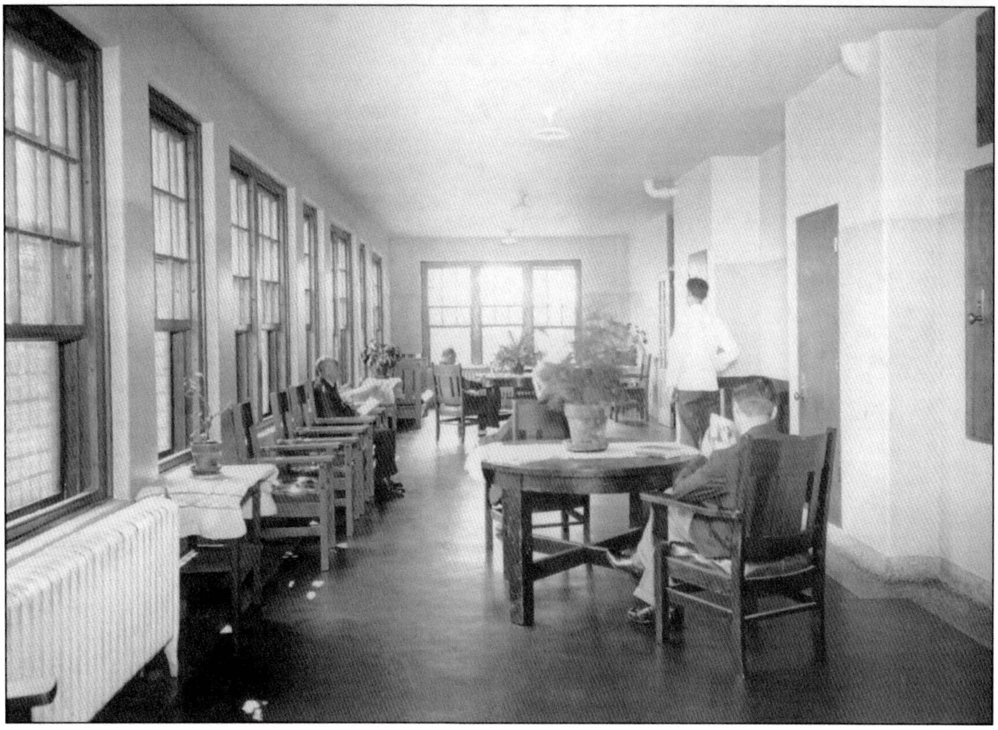

A long dayroom on the male side is depicted here in the 1920s. Activities were limited for most patients at Northampton State Hospital, but here are patients who are fully dressed and engaged in reading, seated on solid furniture in a clean space that is cheered with plants and table runners. This was approximately at the midpoint in the life of the institution.

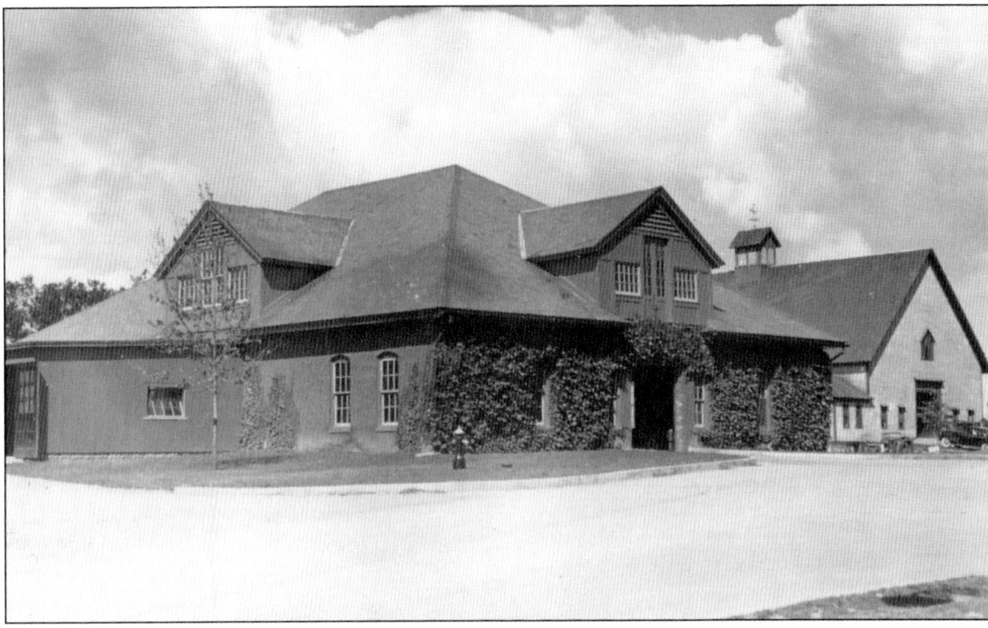

This beautiful brick stable was built in 1900 to house the hospital's driving horses. Stables were located on the main floor with a hayloft above. When automobiles supplanted horses, the stable became a garage after 1922. This building is the oldest hospital structure still extant on the grounds. During the 1998 filming of *Cider House Rules* in the old main building, this barn was used as a screening room. It is now being developed as an animal hospital.

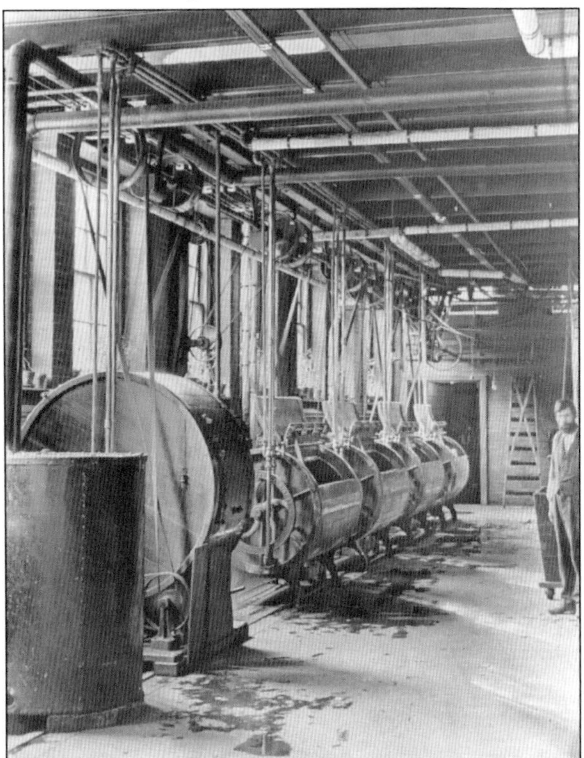

As the hospital grew, the laundry grew with it. After occupying two locations in the back of the main buildings, it moved to this structure in 1913. The laundry was one of the many places, from the wards to the barns and the workshops, where patients worked. When this building was new, it was reported that patients "make tinware, clothing, mattresses, bedding, do all the upholstering, cane seat chairs, do printing, knit garments, make preserves."

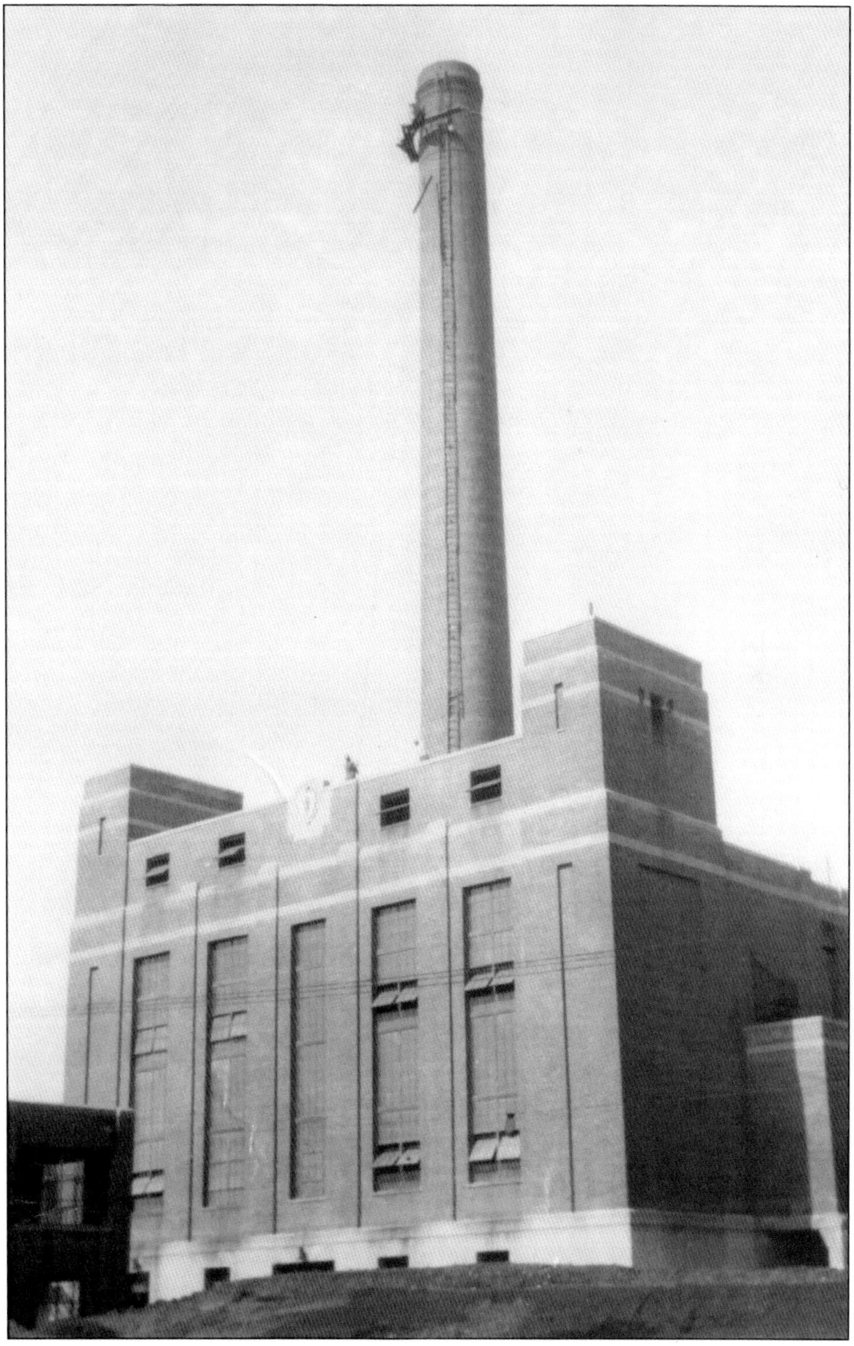

The hospital "should be warmed by passing an abundance of pure fresh air from the external atmosphere, over pipes or plates containing steam under low pressure, or hot water, the temperature of which at the boiler does not exceed 212 degrees F.," and "the boilers for generating steam should be in a detached structure," according to Thomas Kirkbride. The scale of the massive new power plant, built on Earle Street in 1935 as a New Deal construction project, mirrors the enormous size of the hospital. A large power plant increased efficiency and raised output. Sadly, there were no economies of scale in the effective treatment of mental illness.

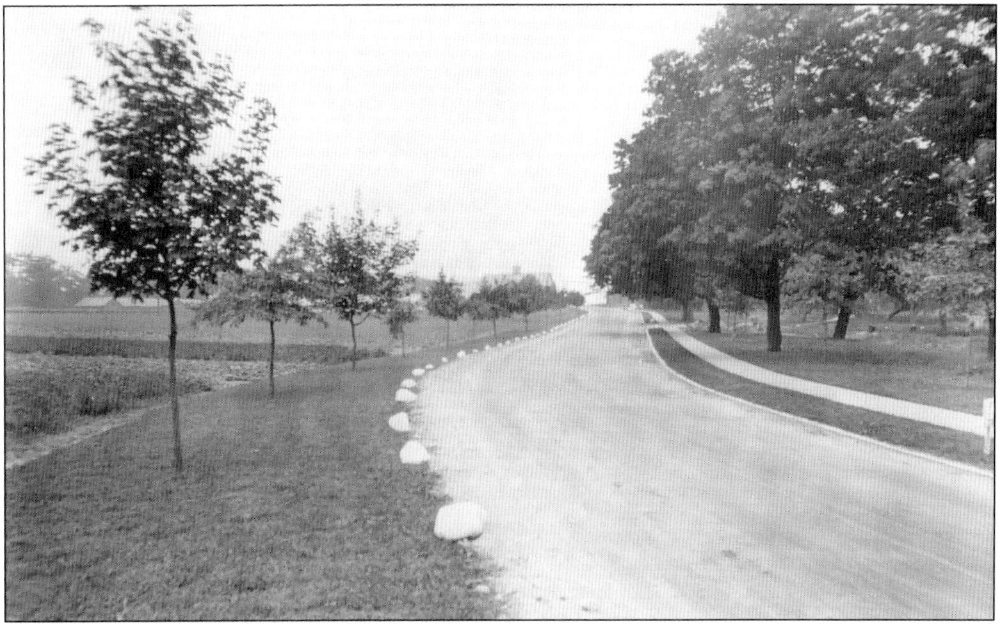

Enormous amounts of vegetables were grown, canned, cooked, and consumed at the hospital. The vegetable fields under cultivation on the farm lands to the west of the main buildings can be seen to the left of the road in this photograph, taken about 1929. That year, more than 160 tons of beans, beets, cabbage, carrots, celery, sweet corn, onions, parsnips, peas, potatoes, pumpkins, squash, tomatoes, turnips, rhubarb, and strawberries were grown in these fields.

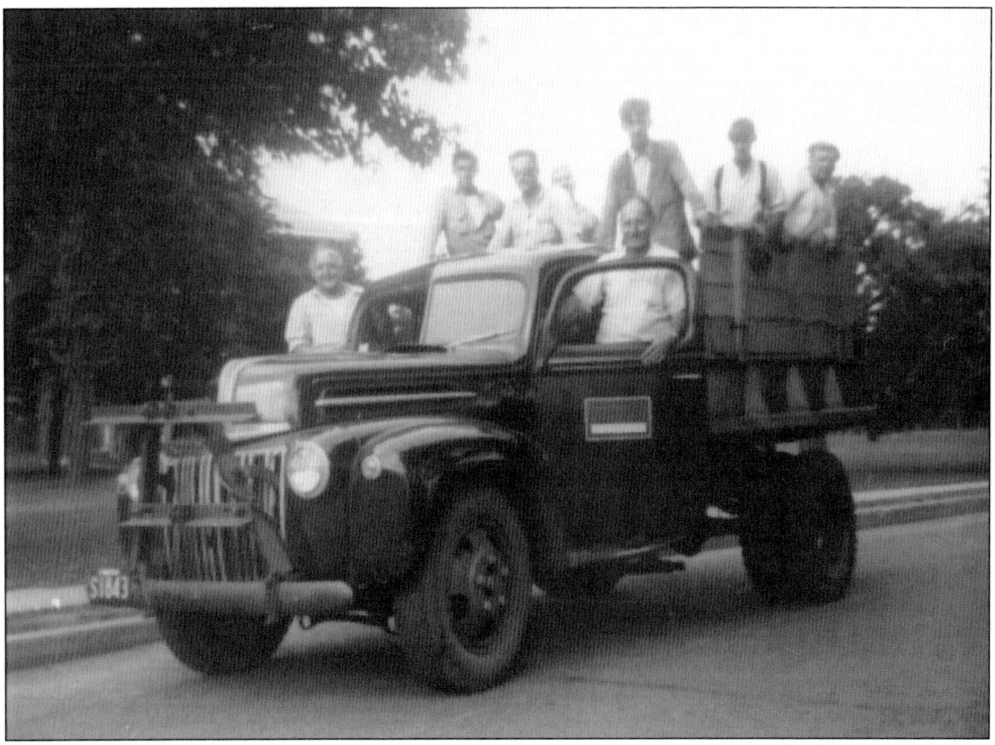

Patient workers ride in the back of the hospital truck driven by employee Charles Musante.

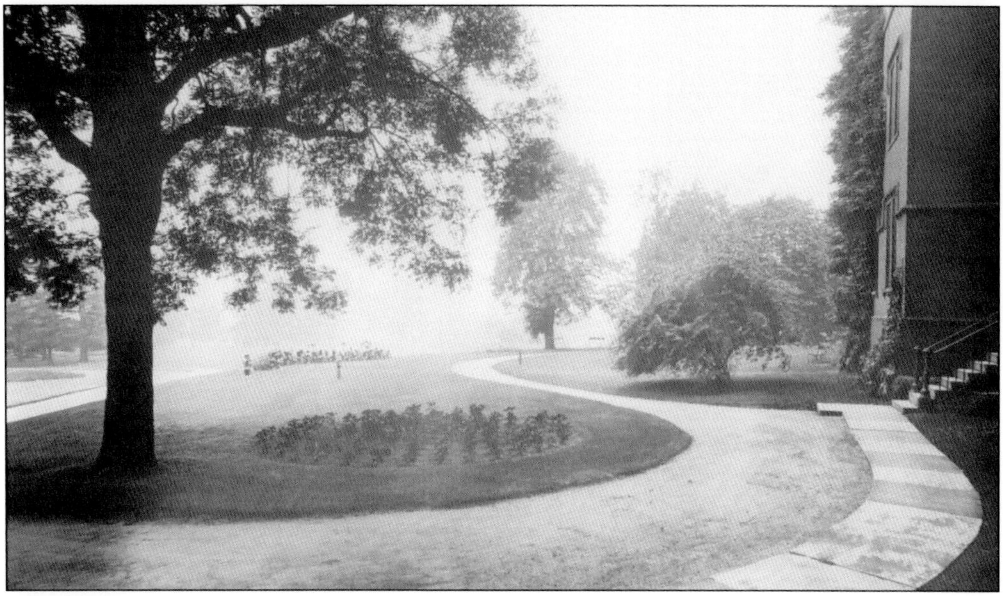

Here is a view of the grounds at the height of their physical beauty, following the ideals of 19th-century moral treatment. "Trees and shrubs, flowering plants, summerhouses, and other pleasing arrangements, add to its attractiveness." The aim for the hospital was to "have a cheerful and comfortable appearance, everything prison-like should be carefully avoided, and the means of effecting the proper degree of security should be masked," according to Thomas Kirkbride's specifications for state hospitals.

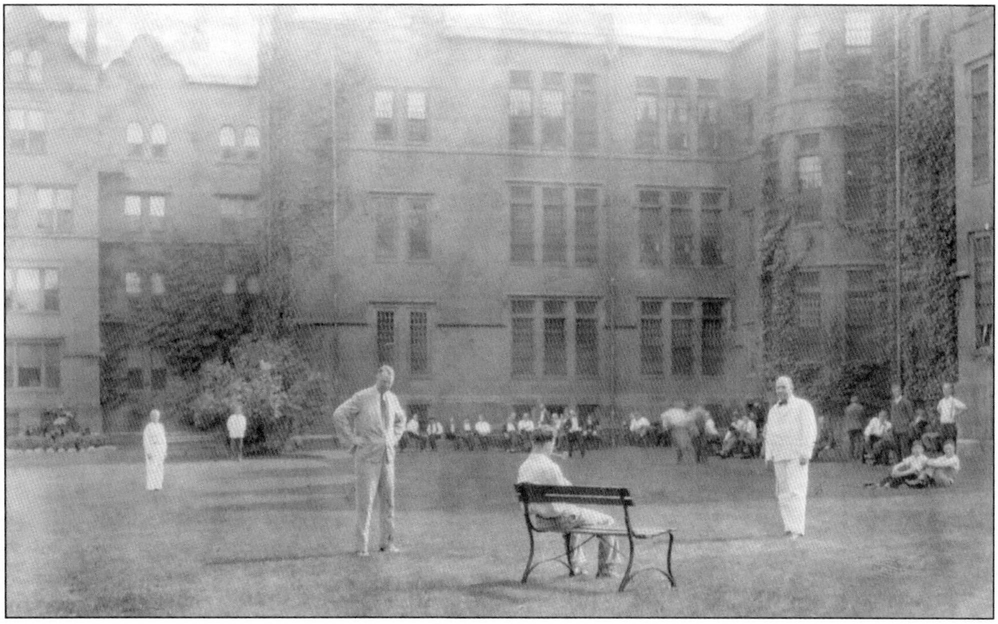

An afternoon scene on the front lawn of the hospital in 1930 offers a rare outdoor glimpse of both buildings and patients. The renovated wards on the north side can be seen with their recently enlarged windows and continuous, ivy-covered walls. Three attendants, dressed in white, stand sentinel over a group of patients while John Gregg, the 6-foot, 7-inch supervisor of male attendants, looms over them all in suit and tie.

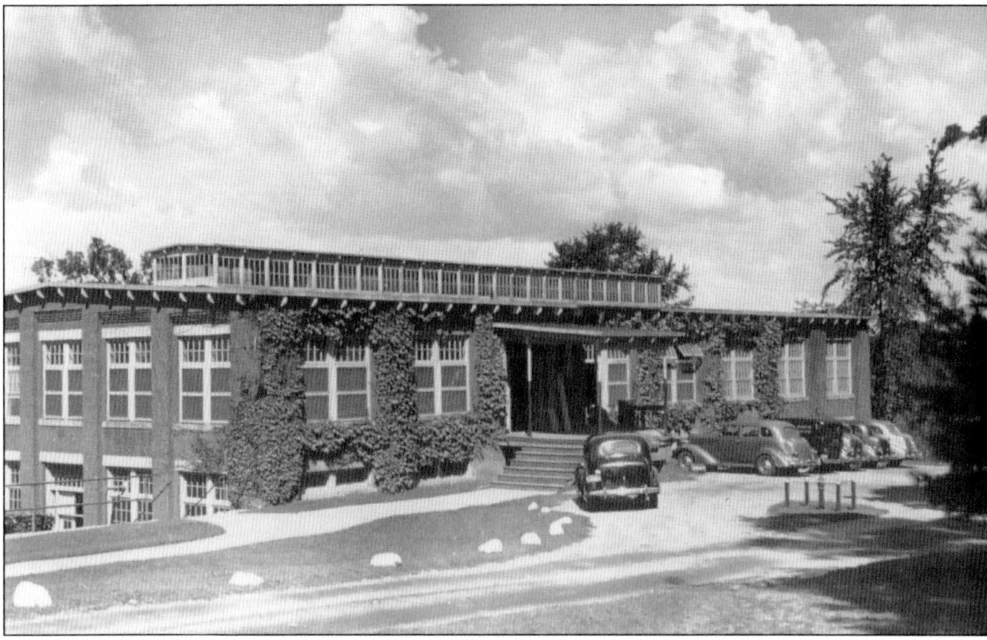

This image evokes a time when the design of both industrial buildings and automobiles showed a pleasing balance of function and beauty. The building was the laundry when new in 1913. That use was supplanted by the large utilitarian structure built on Earle Road in 1936. This building became the carpentry shop, serving for that purpose in the ensuing decades.

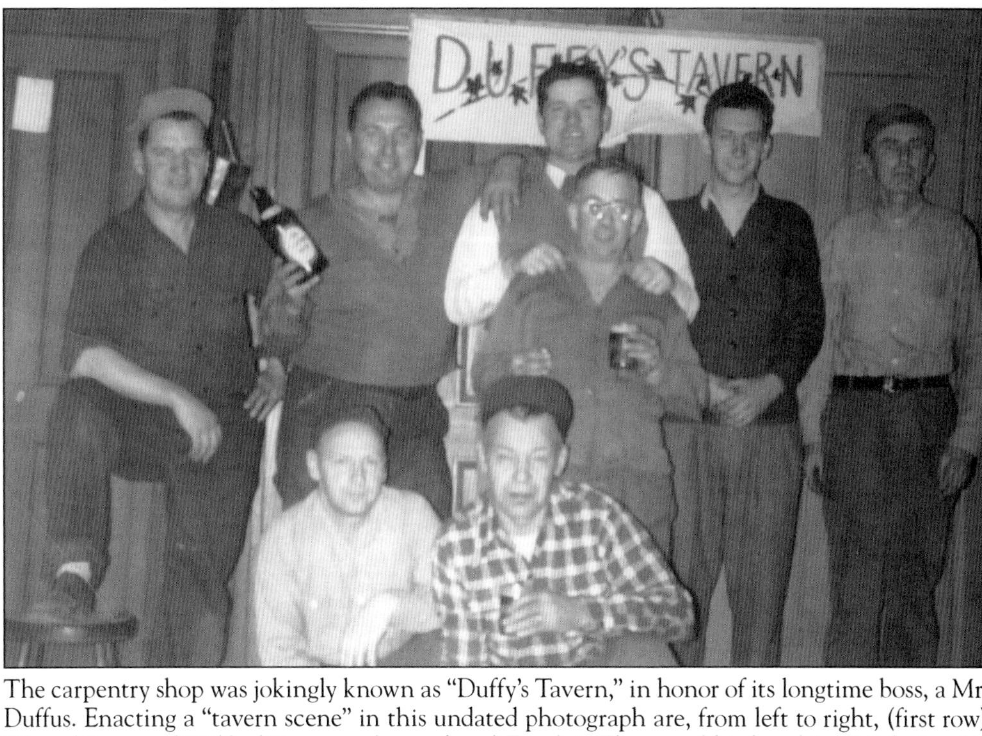

The carpentry shop was jokingly known as "Duffy's Tavern," in honor of its longtime boss, a Mr. Duffus. Enacting a "tavern scene" in this undated photograph are, from left to right, (first row) Edward Press and Wilfred Turcotte; (second row) Frank LaFlamme; (third row) Joe Michalowski, Frank Misterka, George Hyde, Robert Norotny, and Joe Reardon.

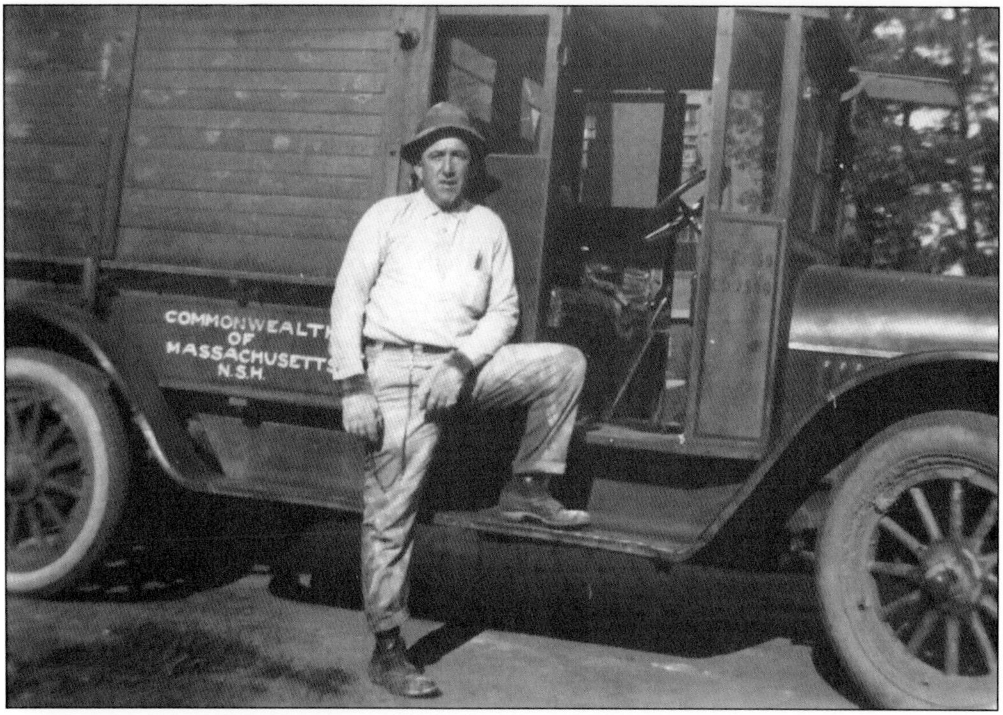

Carmi Harte, above, worked on the hospital farm for many years before taking over the salvage yard. His daughter and stepdaughter both had long and successful careers working at the hospital. Francis McCarthy (below left) was an attendant who rose to become the chief supervisor of the male side in the 1950s. With him are, from left to right, Bill Warnock, who worked at the hospital for 40 years, first on the farm and then as chauffeur to the medical staff; Jim Musante, who ran the piggery; and his wife, Dot, who was an attendant and then worked in the clothes-marking department. Together, these four put in more than 100 years on the job and were related by blood or marriage to dozens of other hospital employees.

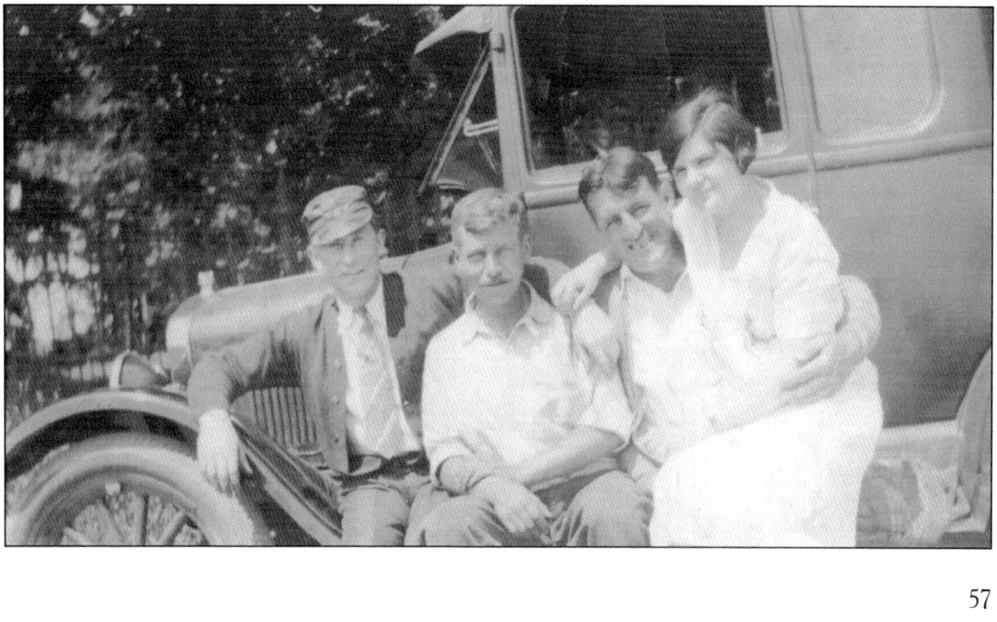

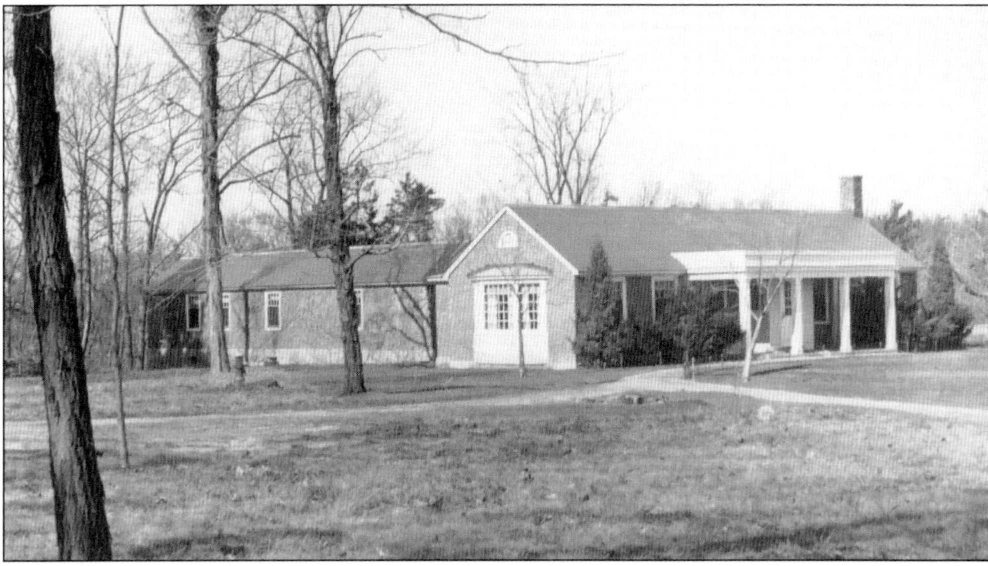

During the day, patients with privileges could play cards, shoot billiards, smoke, or buy candy and drinks at the clubhouse. At night, employees used it for their bowling leagues. Treasurer Elizabeth Provost met her future husband, Leo, while bowling. It was built in 1932 to replace an earlier club that had burned down in 1922.

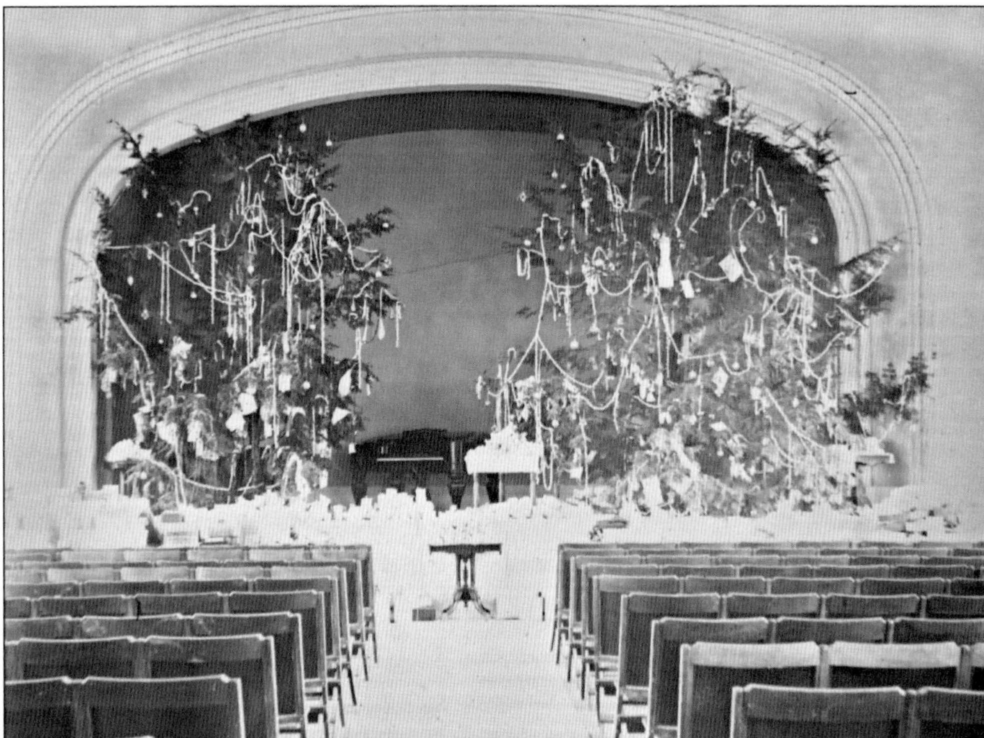

Christmas is being celebrated at the hospital about 1900. Trees have been mounted and decorated in the new chapel. Some patients have knitted mittens and caps that are hung on the tree as gifts for others.

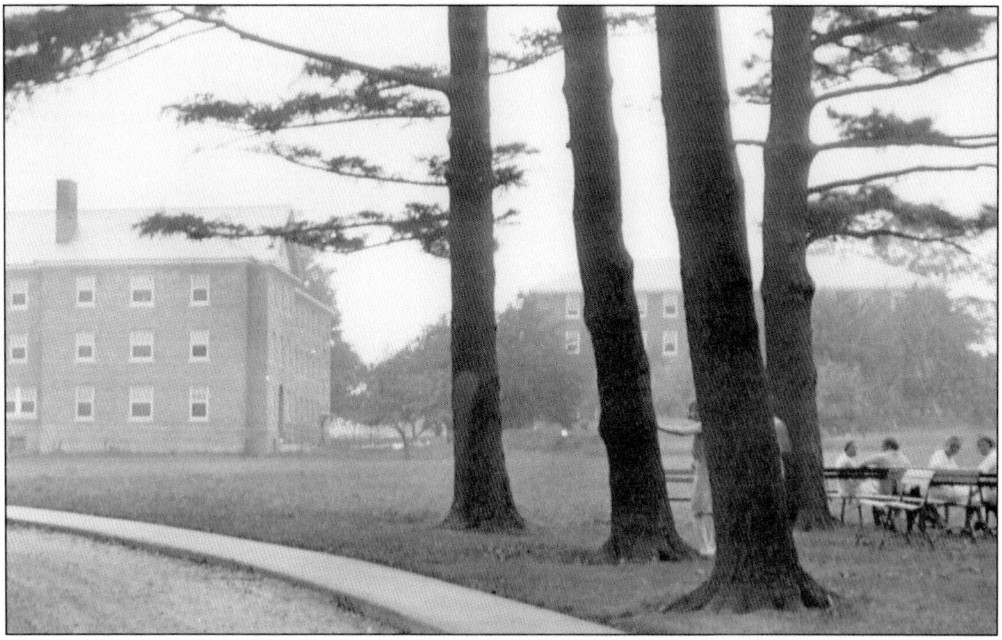

This atmospheric view shows patients making use of the grounds on the edge of a grove of trees. The Nurses' Home, at left, and South Home loom in the background.

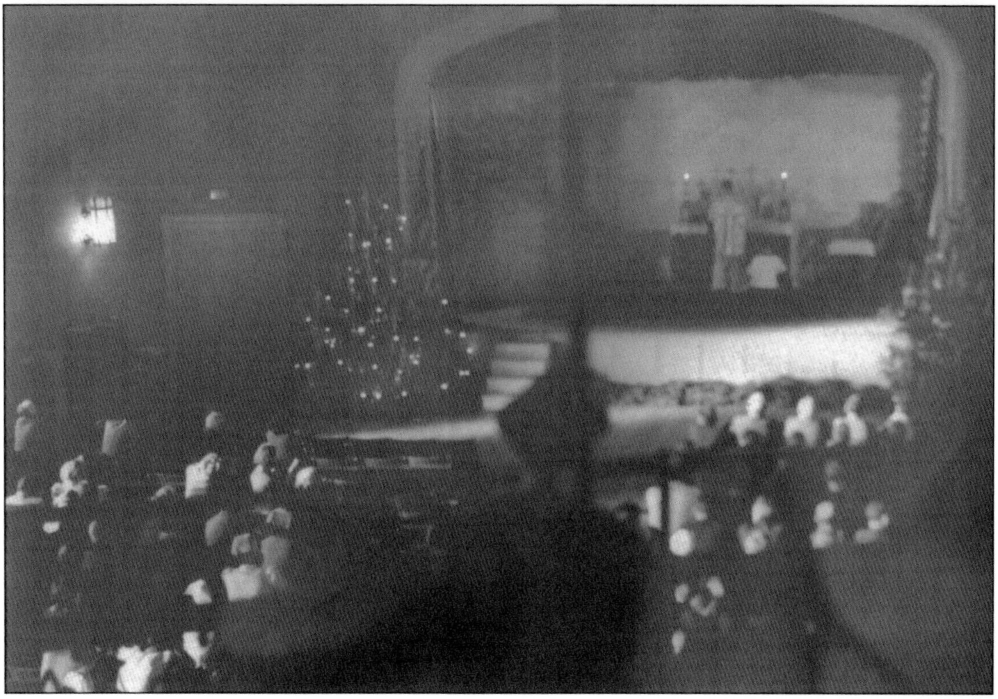

The bylaws of the hospital required weekly religious services: "Indeed is not the proposition both plausible and reasonable that such an institution should be made a microcosm in itself—a little world within which men and women shall find as many as possible of those sources of rational enjoyment to which they were formerly accustomed," wrote Supt. Pliny Earle in 1866. Here, Christmas Mass is being celebrated.

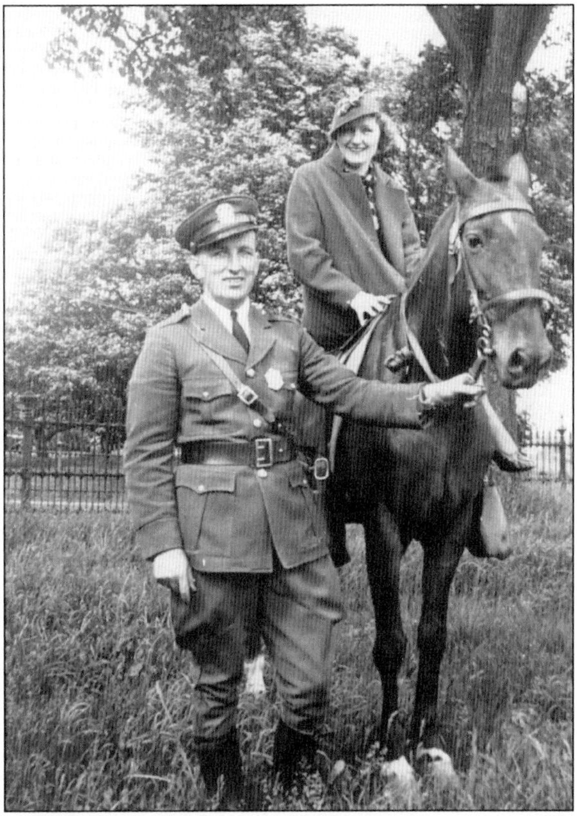

Attendant Molly McCarthy gets a ride on the horse of hospital security officer Jim Coffey. The iron fence that enclosed the hospital grounds since the 1870s was ripped out and donated to a scrap metal drive during World War II.

The hospital baseball team, comprised of employees, poses for a picture in the early 1930s. NSH played teams from local factories and businesses, other state hospitals, and even the Springfield Police Department. In 1939, they played 47 games with an average attendance of 475 patients per game. Richard Frennier, first row at left, was the captain and also the head attendant for the male wards.

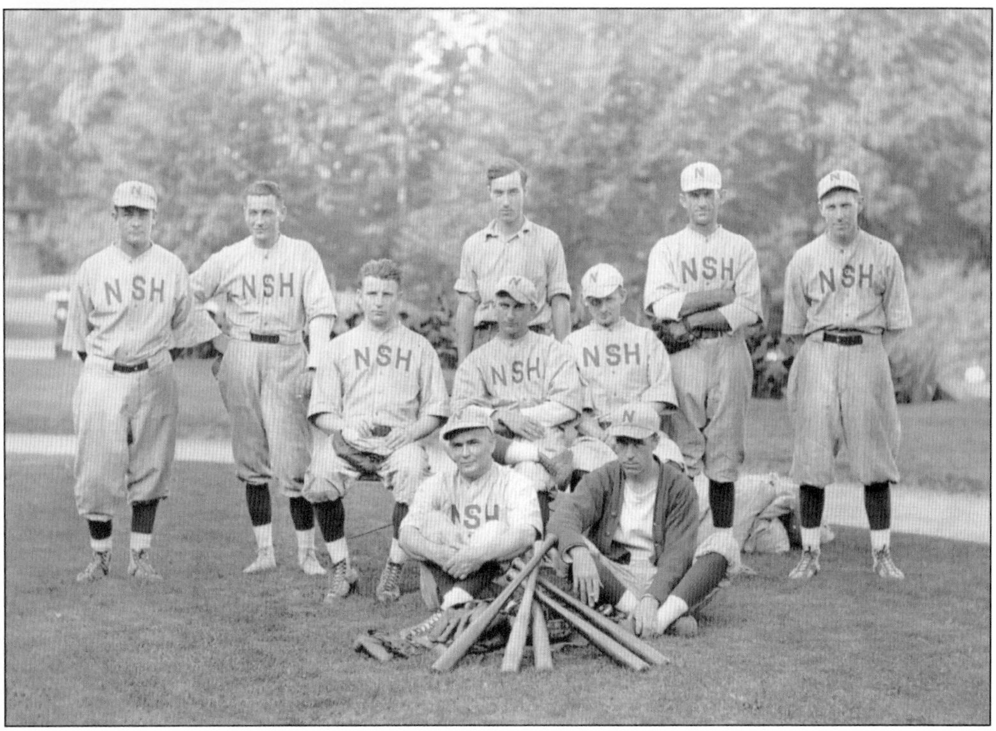

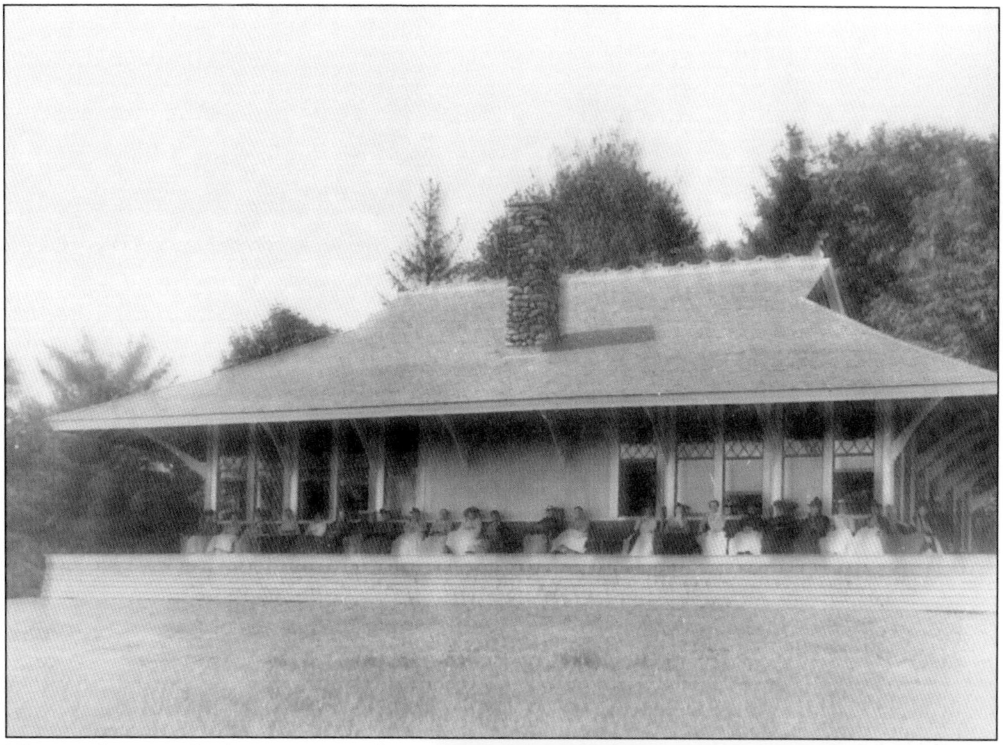

The pavilion was built in 1898, a gift from Martha Eastman of Amherst in memory of her sister who was a patient at the hospital. "Knowing that the Commonwealth provides liberally the necessary buildings for the care of those who must come here, and realizing how great a part diversion plays in the treatment of their disordered intellects, she felt it her privilege to provide for their pleasure a pavilion," noted the superintendent in the annual report. George Button Sr., pictured at right, worked in the power plant. He is seen relaxing on the built-in bench at the pavilion. The handsome architectural details of this 1898 building are revealed.

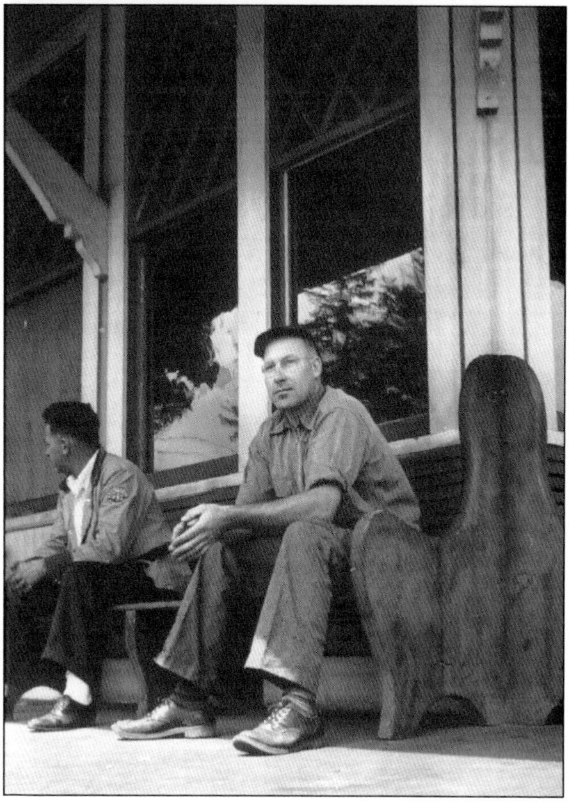

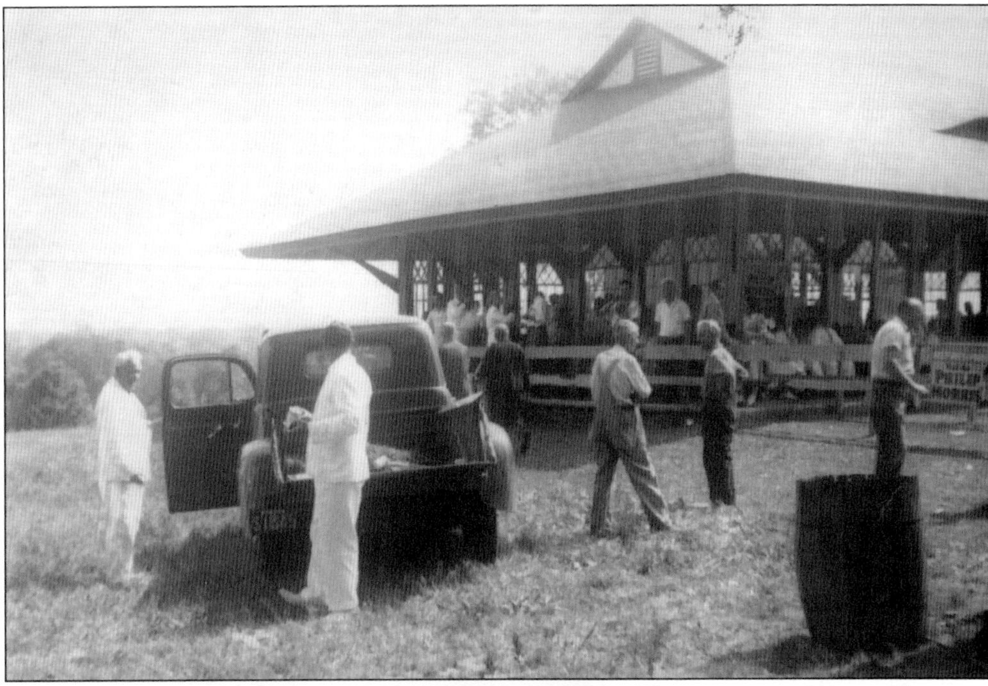

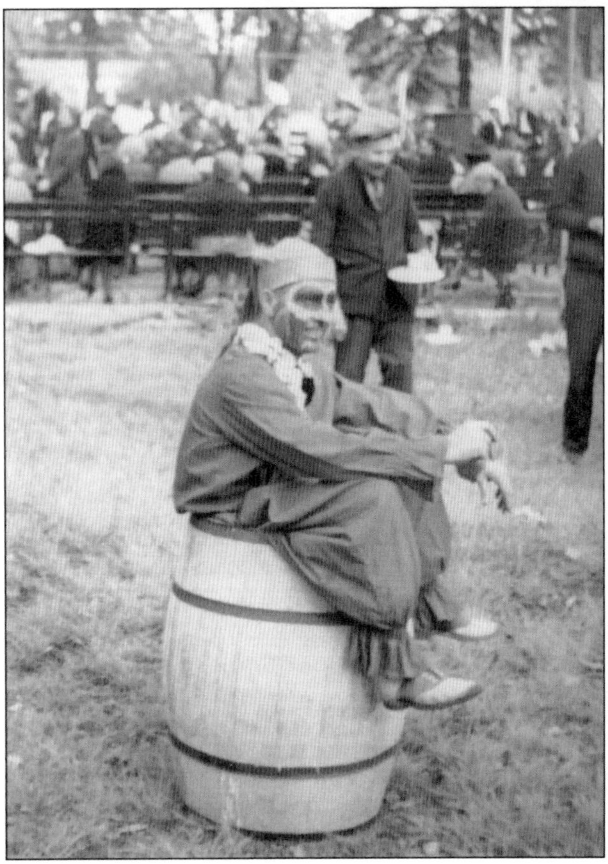

The patients and the staff mingled freely in the outdoors on occasions such as this—a rare departure from the control on the wards that was a constant of hospital life. When the hospital confined 2,500 people with a wide variety of problems, behaviors, and needs, the requirements of the institution for order and regimentation became paramount. This came at the cost of freedom of choice and movement for the majority of individual patients.

On the first annual field day in 1935, more than 1,500 of the 2,200 patients resident at the hospital were brought outside for a day of festivities. For some, this was the first time they had left the locked wards in years. Picnic lunches were served near the pavilion. Performing acts entertained on a makeshift stage. Attendant Dominic Mazilli is the clown in the barrel.

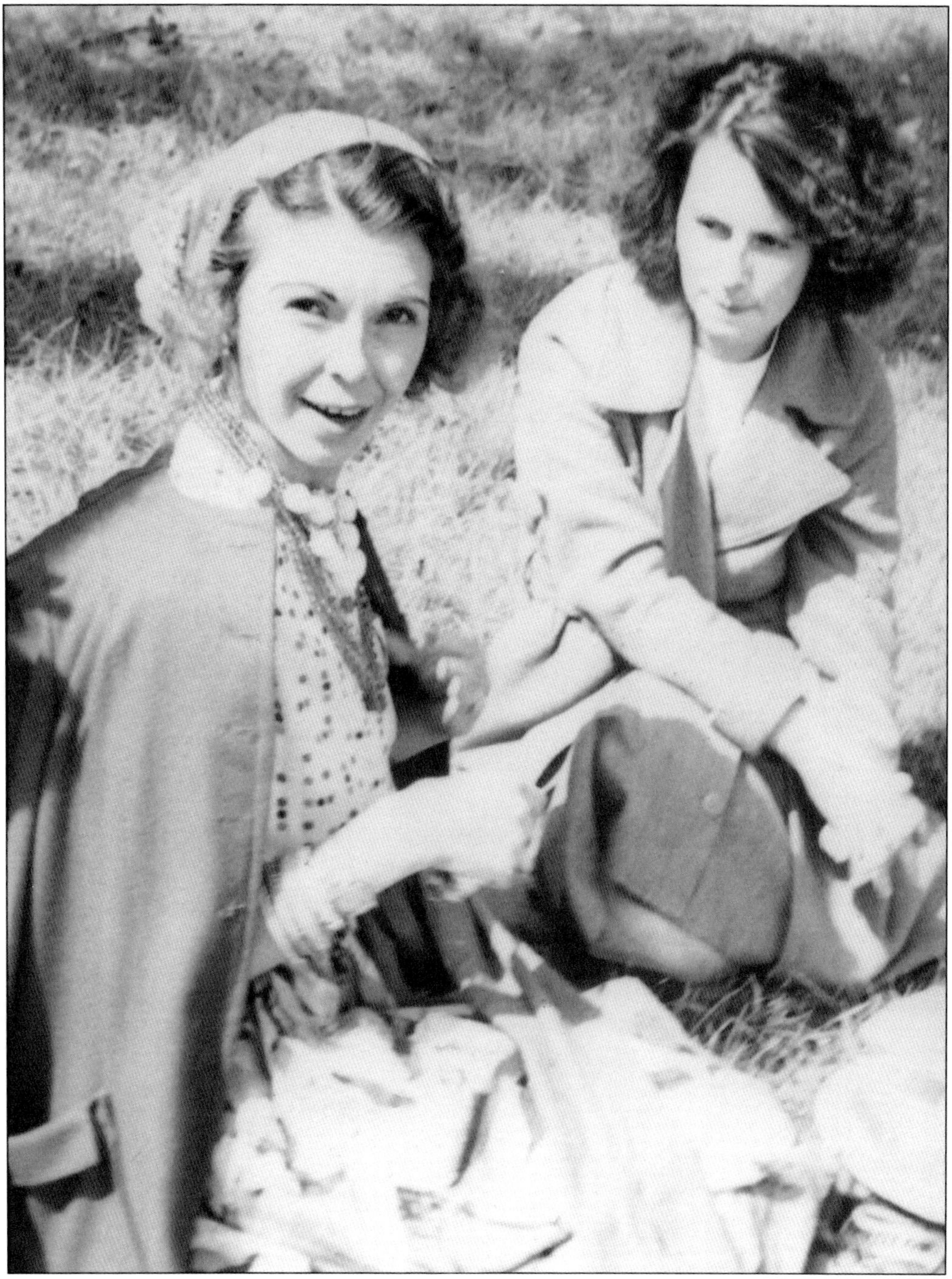

Field day must have been a welcome and exciting change from the monotony and constriction of daily life on the wards for patients at the hospital. Employee Betty Barnes, left, and an unidentified woman, believed to be a patient, sit together on the lawn during field day in 1940. Barnes may be telling the young woman's fortune with the help of tarot cards.

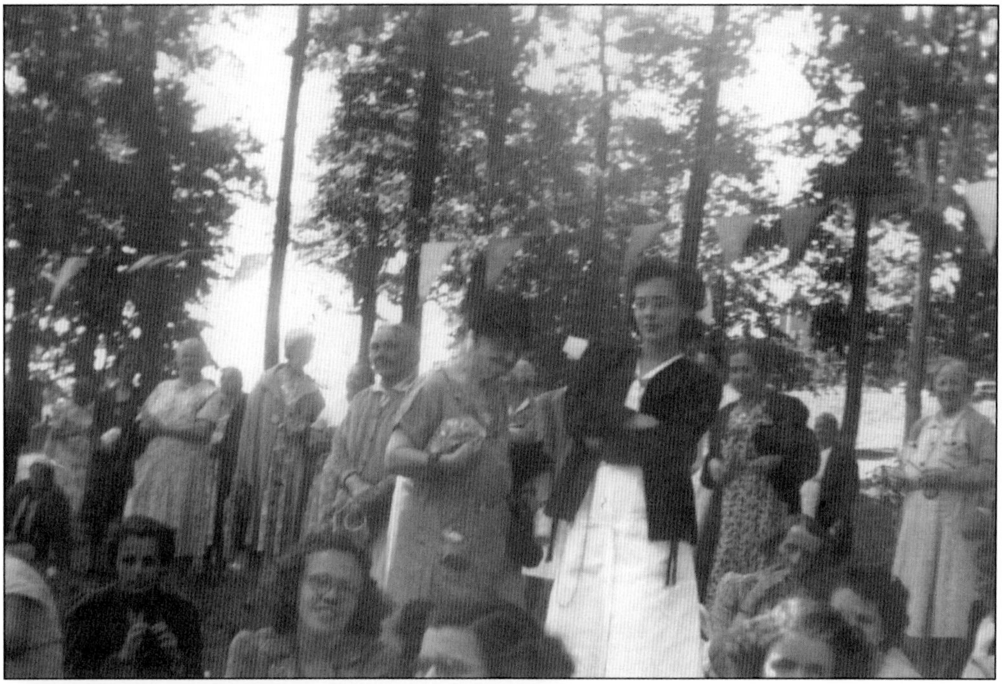

Nurse Glenna McLaughlin watches field day events with unidentified patients in the late 1930s. At this time, the average length of stay of patients in the hospital was more than 8.5 years. While many patients grew old at the hospital, many more were admitted when old. In 1936, one third of first admissions were more than 60 years old. A total of 147 patients died in the hospital that year, and half were older than 70.

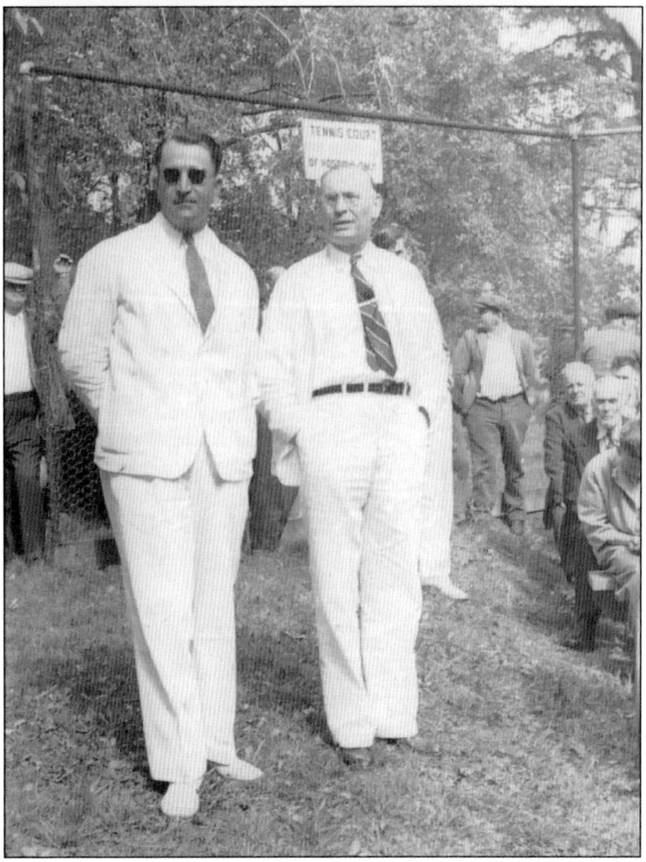

The entire hospital staff worked on field day. Hundreds of patients who seldom or never left their wards were brought out to the expansive lawns in front of the main buildings. Here, attendants Alphonse Gregory, left, and Henry Loiselle stand amidst unidentified patients on field day in 1936.

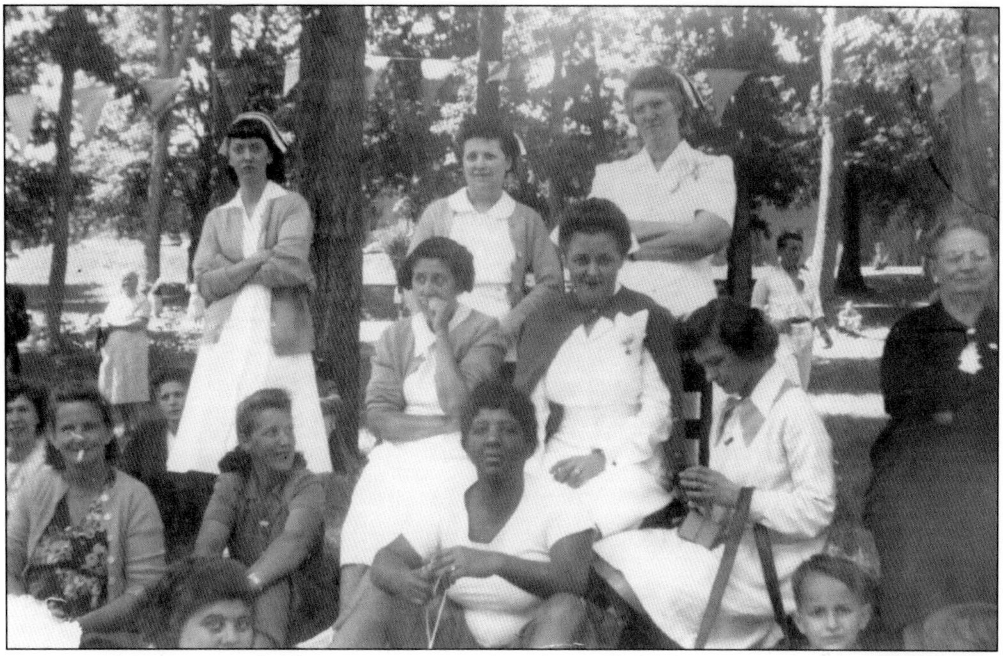

Nurses and patients and a few guests sit together during field day activities around 1936. The patients and children are unidentified. From left to right, the standing nurses are unidentified, Barbara Gilligan, and Minnie Ducharme Hayward. Sitting are, from left to right, ? Brassil and Marion Packard. Kay Grigsby kneels to the right of Packard.

Starting in 1928, patient care buildings were erected across Prince Street from the main buildings on land purchased 50 years earlier by Pliny Earle, who spoke of it as "commanding a view that can scarcely be equaled in Western Massachusetts." By 1936, there were four buildings with 12 wards as well as a separate dining commons. These wards were used primarily for the housing of chronic, long-term patients.

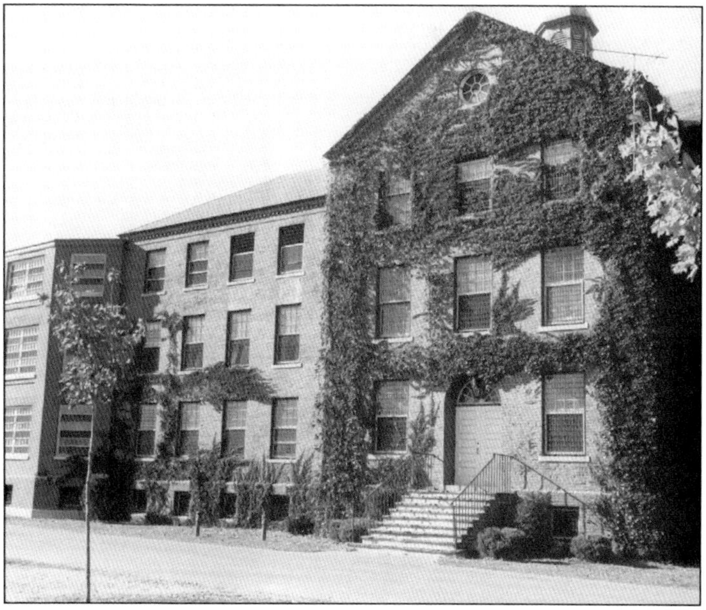

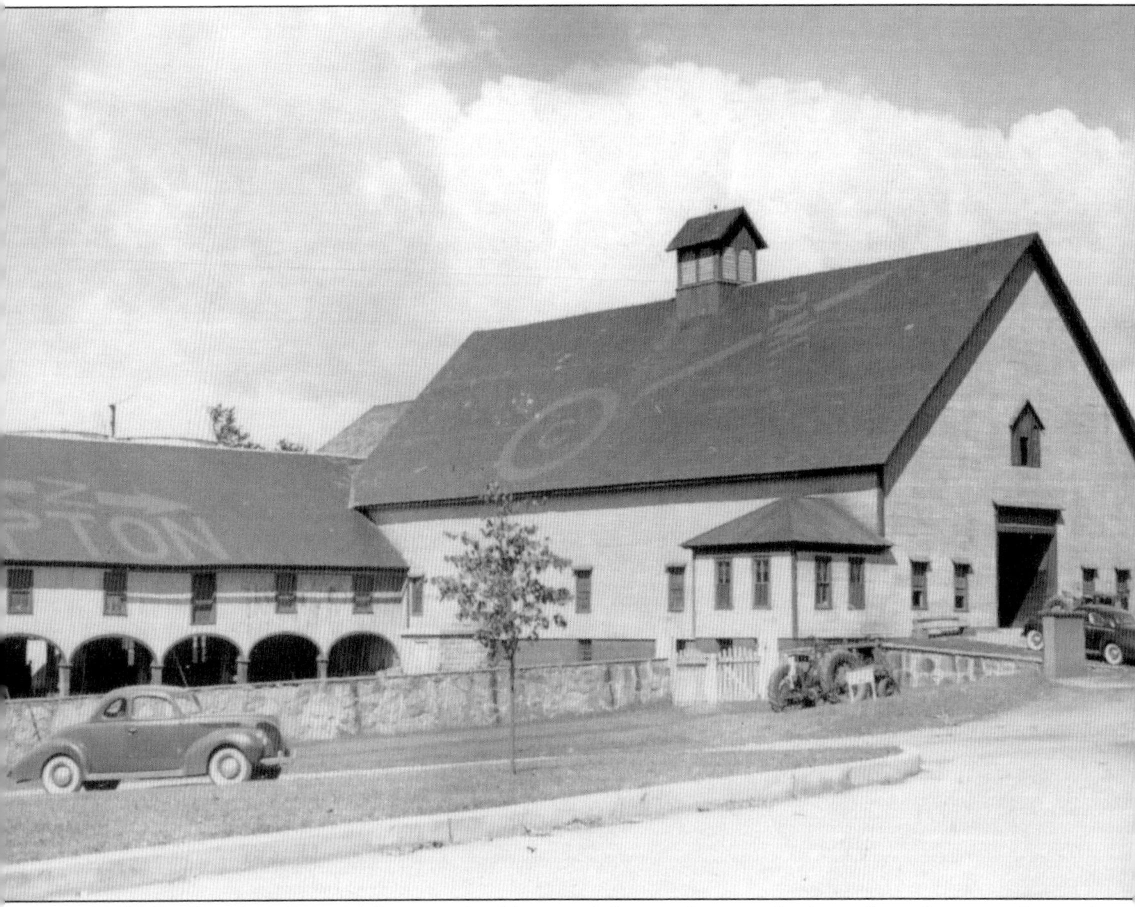

The big barn just behind the main building and the pavilion on the large front lawn was burned to the ground one day in 1960. The superintendent had been warning since 1945 of the fire hazard the barn represented. Elizabeth "Betty" Provost, the institutional treasurer, witnessed the fire and later described it this way: "All over the neighborhood the menfolk converged to let out the livestock and help with the patients. The barn was full of baled hay and went up in a cloud of black smoke that was visible for miles, sparks falling all over creation."

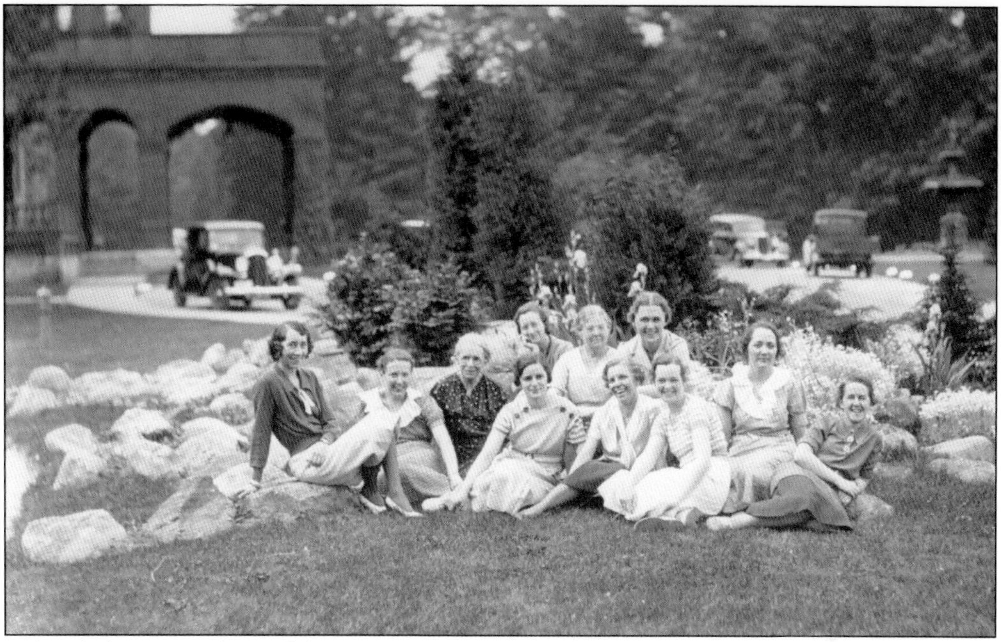

Relaxed charm in a beautiful setting is an unexpected surprise in photographs of the hospital. Treasurer Eva Graves, by appearance and by many accounts a hard taskmaster, is surrounded by the office clerical staff in this 1935 photograph.

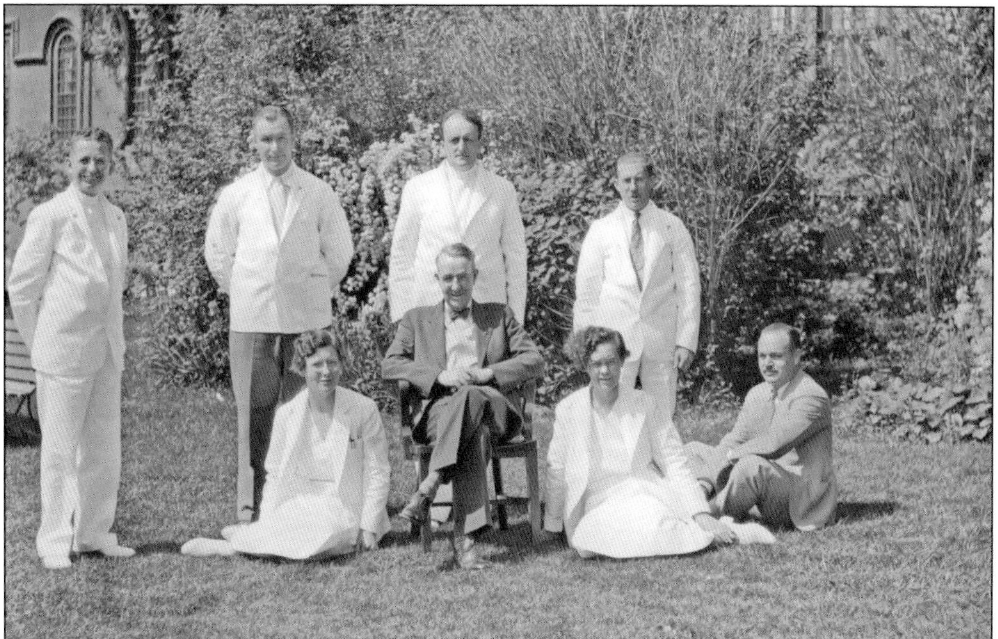

Newly appointed superintendent Arthur N. Ball is surrounded by his medical staff in this 1935 portrait. Dr. Ball trained at Northampton and served on the medical staff from 1912 to 1921. When he returned, he was quick to initiate new policies, including the opening of some wards during the day to give patients free access to the grounds. He organized field day in his first year. During Ball's tenure, new medical treatments, such as electroconvulsive therapy, were introduced.

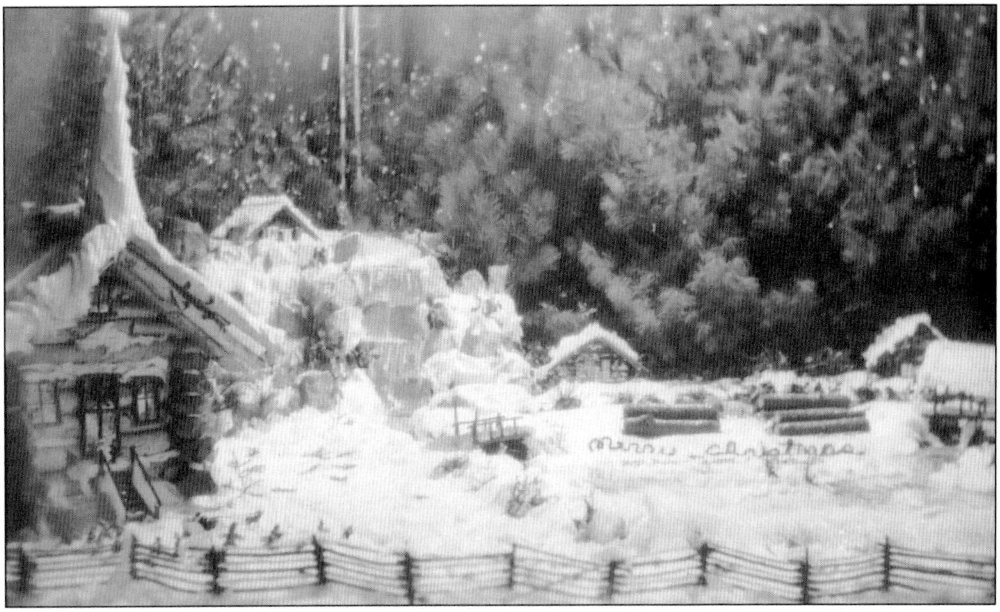

In 1935, Charles Searles of the occupational therapy department created this beautiful Christmas display on the first floor of the first ward on the north side of the hospital. The male patients on this ward, which was the closest to the main entrance, were "of the better grade" as regards to their behavior. Most worked at the hospital and all had grounds privileges.

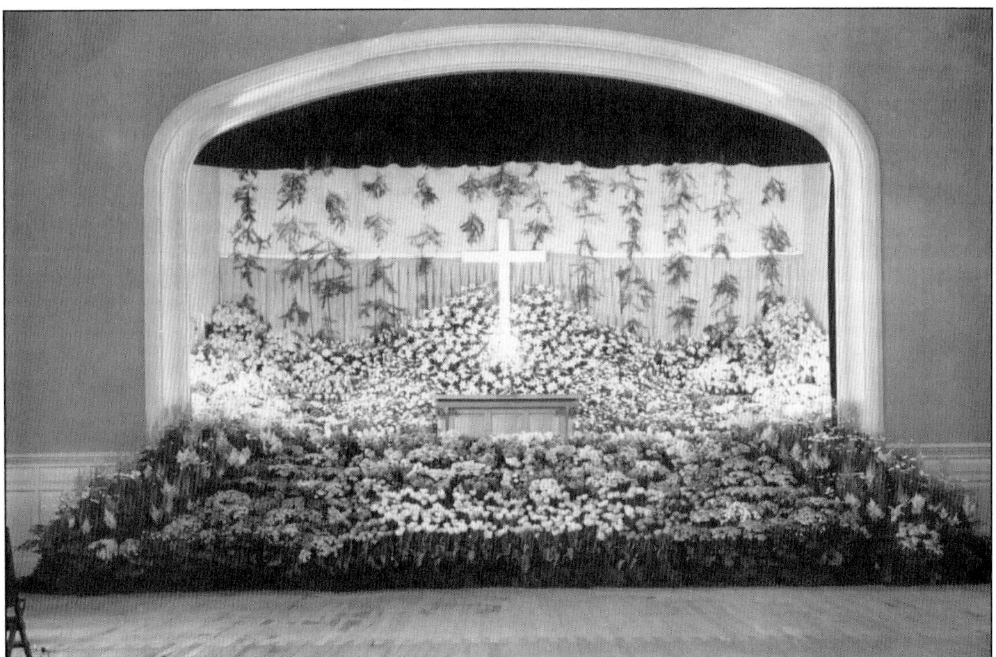

For Easter, the chapel was decorated with plants grown in the hospital greenhouse. A total of 852 tulip and lily plants adorned the chapel in this photograph from 1939. The display was enjoyed by 1,500 visitors over the weekend and brightened the wards in the following weeks. The joyful abundance of these decorations stayed in the memory of many who saw it, long after the hospital closed.

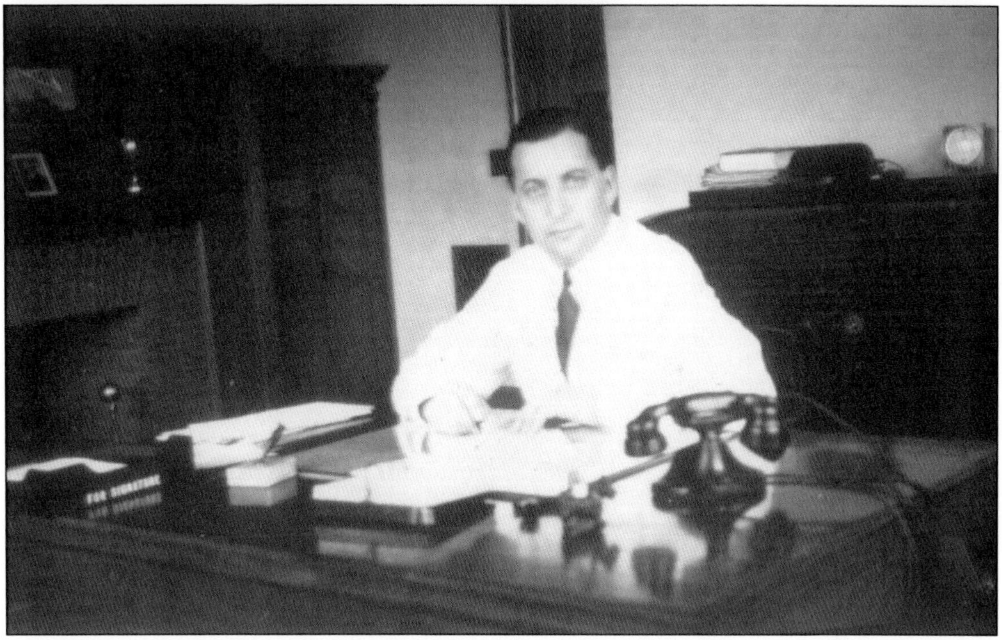

Latvian-born and German-educated Dr. Harry Michelson was the clinical director at the hospital for 10 years. He resigned to go into private practice in 1952. It was reported that he felt thwarted in efforts to create a more dynamic approach in the treatment of the patients by a system that included many physicians untrained in psychiatry, patient overcrowding and staff shortages, and a general attitude that custodial care was a sufficient goal.

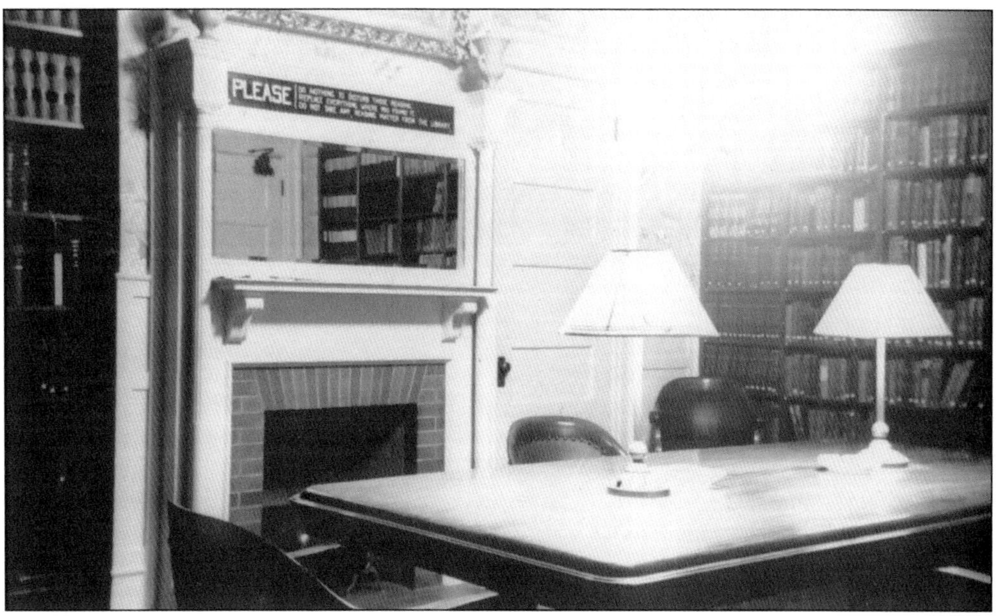

A medical library was maintained in the main building. Pliny Earle set a high intellectual standard in the early years of the hospital. In the 1950s, it was noted that it had become hard to attract young doctors interested in deploying the latest knowledge in their field because Northampton was remote from the centers of training and research.

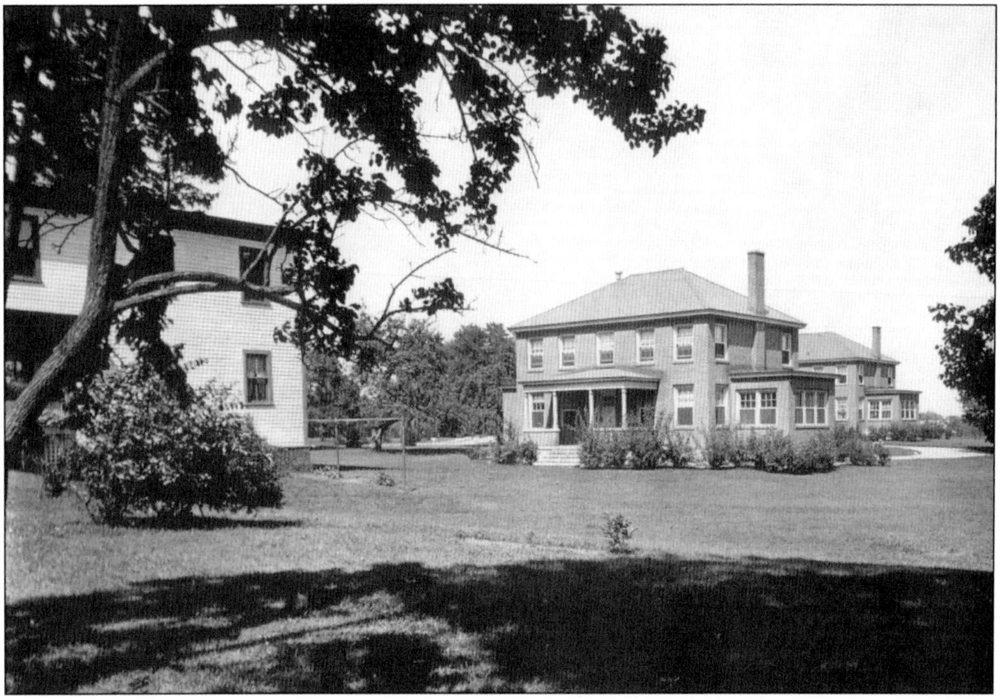

These houses stood near the main entrance on Prince Street. The clapboard house on the left, built before 1853, was the home of George Ellsworth, whose farm was purchased to build the asylum. It served as the home of head farmer John Mercier until his death in 1911. In the early 1970s, it housed the Mental Patients' Advocacy Project, a groundbreaking, federally funded program to train paralegals to advocate for the patients. This was the group that brought the class-action suit that eventually closed the hospital. The brick homes, built in 1928, were home to the steward and an assistant physician.

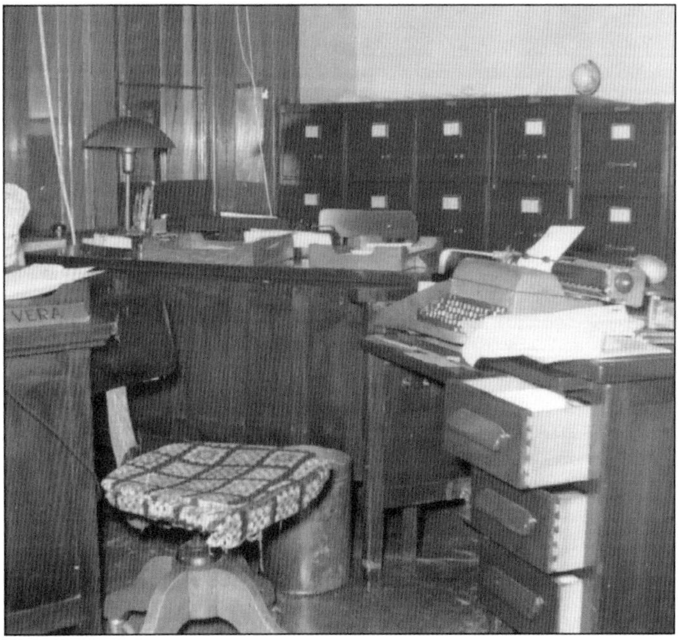

Vera Frennier was the principal clerk for many years, working for the superintendent and overseeing a clerical staff. Several worked crammed in this office in the main building.

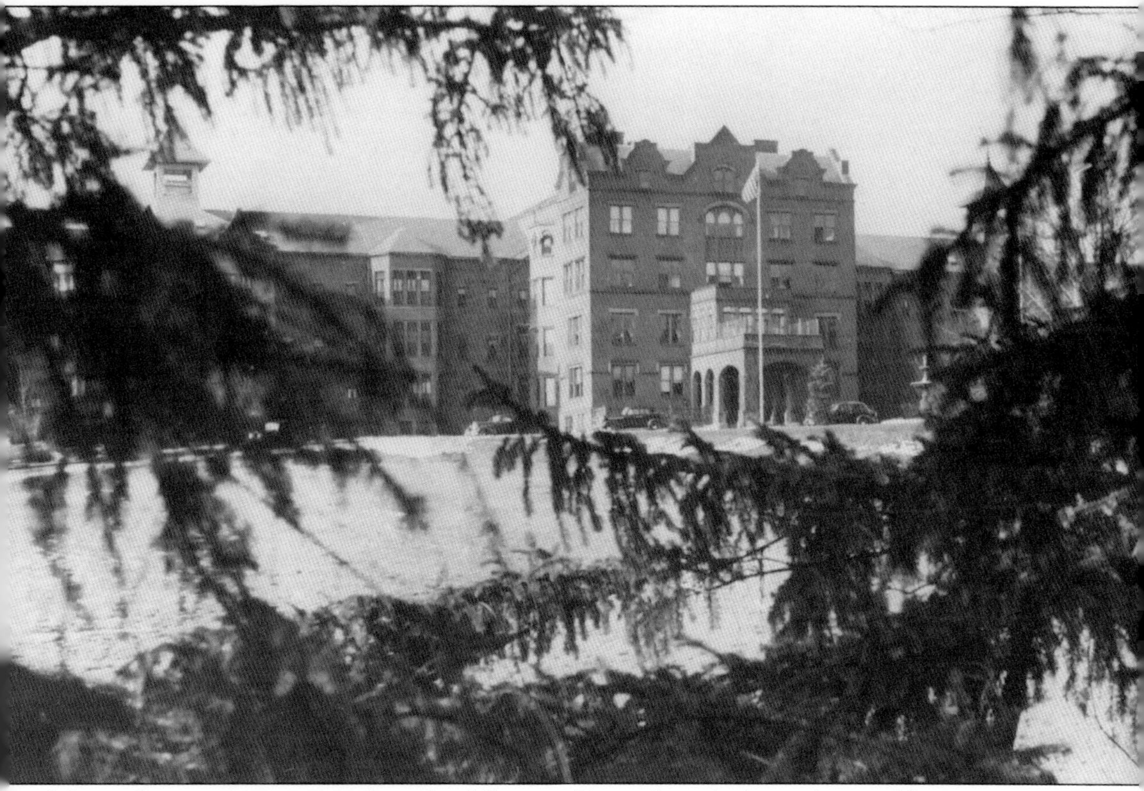

John, a former patient, remembers the following: "At night at bedtime the ward became very silent, and depending where you slept you were able to hear the staff members leave the state hospital, get in their cars talking to each other, start their cars and drive off. Over in the main old building in my bedroom I heard them every night. After they left everything went real quiet, and then you would hear the keys of the night charge nurse entering the ward. The first thing that would pop in my mind was, damn, I hate this place."

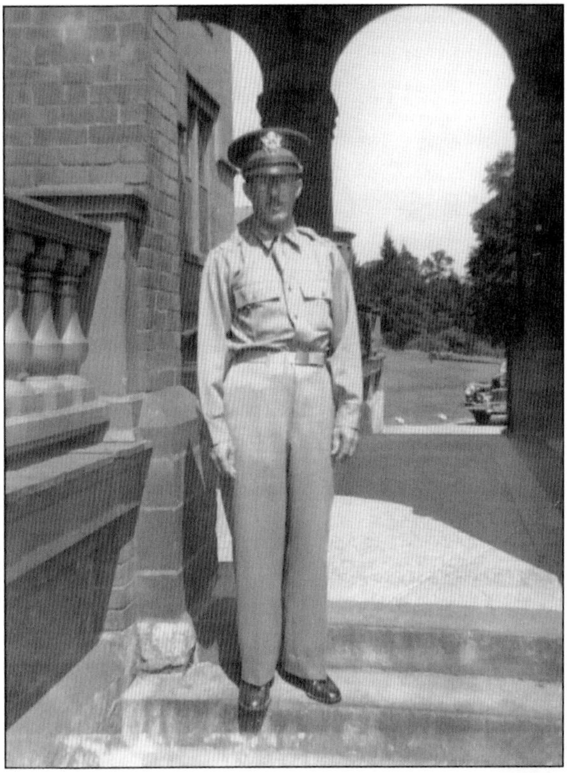

Dr. Guy Randall came to the hospital as assistant superintendent in 1934. He served in the US Army in World War II. The war had a far-reaching impact on mental health care in America, as a new consensus began to develop that early identification of symptoms and treatment in community settings could head off the need for prolonged stays in a hospital. This outlook would divert interest from the state hospitals, which were, until this time, the entire focus of public mental health care.

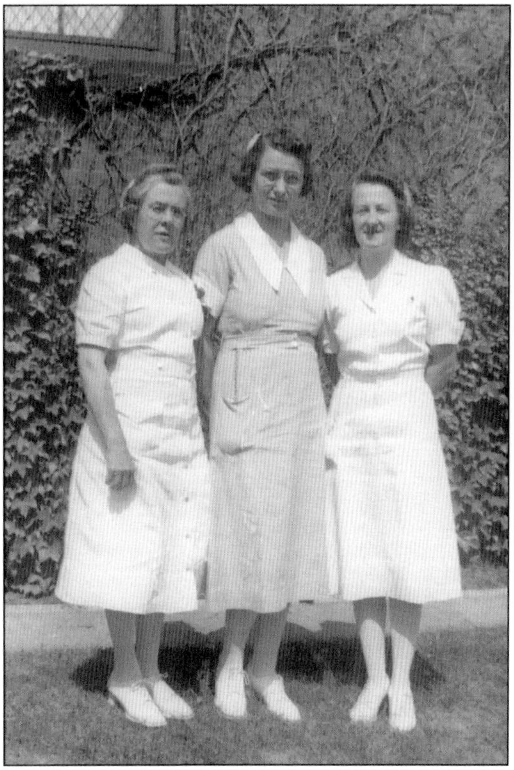

While there was enormous turnover of staff at the hospital, there were also many who worked for decades there. On the left is Sarah Sharpe McCrillis, 25 years after her nurse's training, still working at the hospital in 1940 (she appears as a young trainee on pages 23–25). In the center stands attendant Erna Meckel. The nurse on the right is unidentified.

A long-term employee remembers, "People were brought in for nothing, believe me. If you didn't like what your wife did you could have her pink-slipped, and the police would come to your house and take her. And then you stayed here." This winter photograph of the main entrance reminds the viewer of the many-layered history of this institution—ideally, as a place of refuge for those seeking treatment, and at its worst, a custodial institution without outlet.

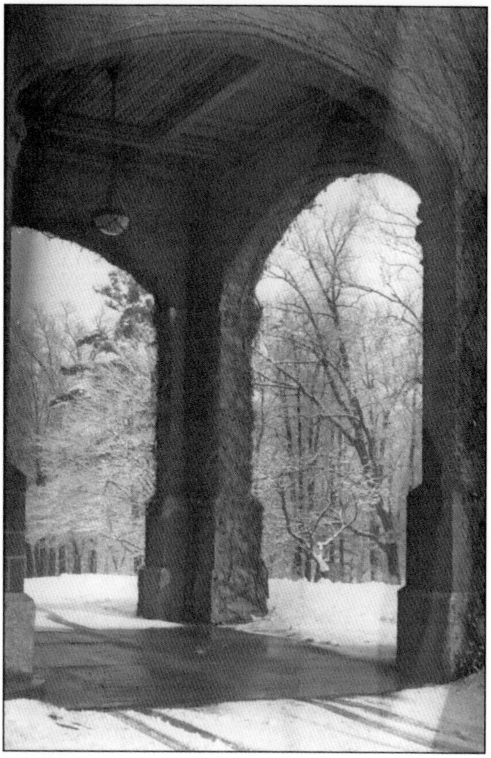

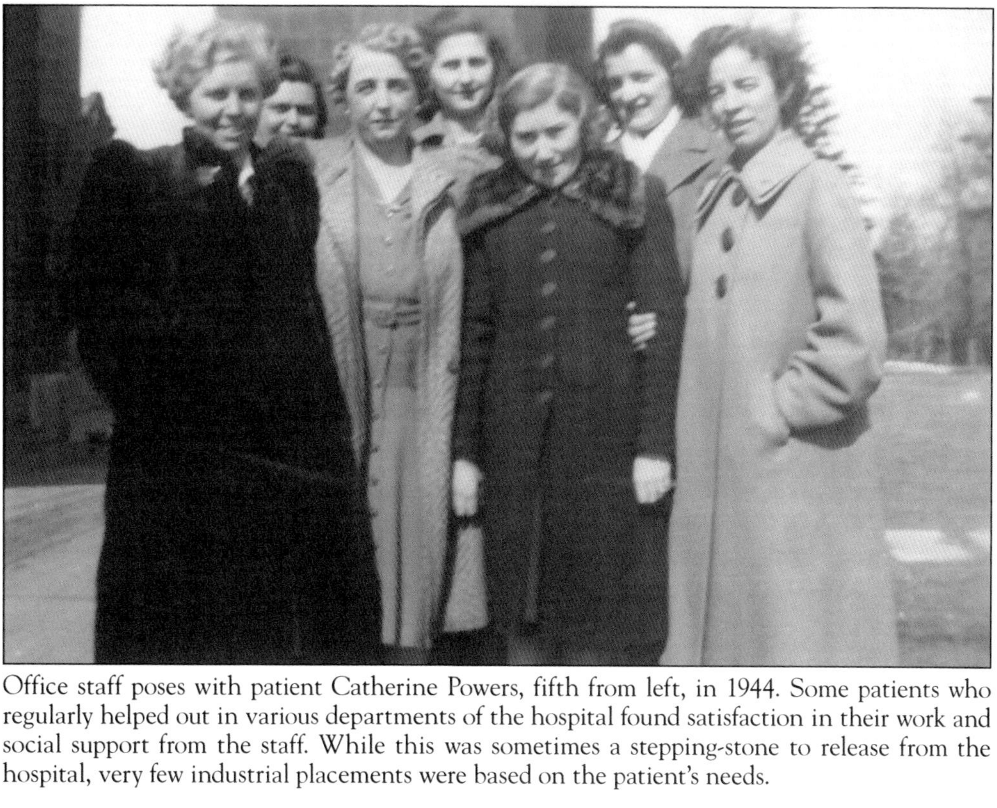

Office staff poses with patient Catherine Powers, fifth from left, in 1944. Some patients who regularly helped out in various departments of the hospital found satisfaction in their work and social support from the staff. While this was sometimes a stepping-stone to release from the hospital, very few industrial placements were based on the patient's needs.

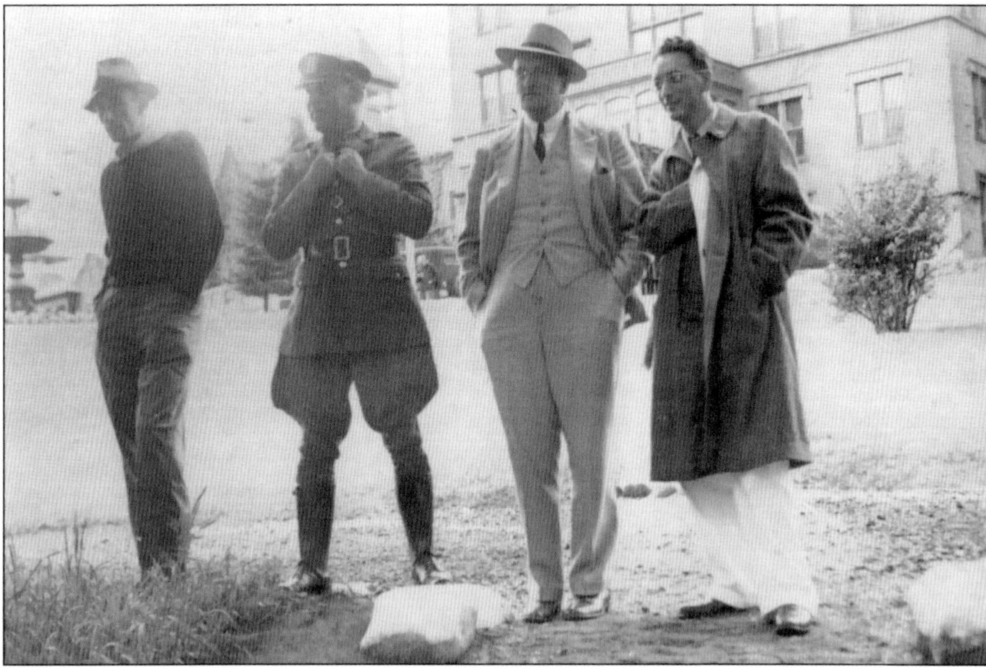

These two photographs were snapped within moments of each other in front of the main building about 1940. The men are, from right to left, assistant physician Phillip Shapiro, assistant superintendent Fernand Longpre, officer Patrick Connors, and unidentified. All of the women are unidentified.

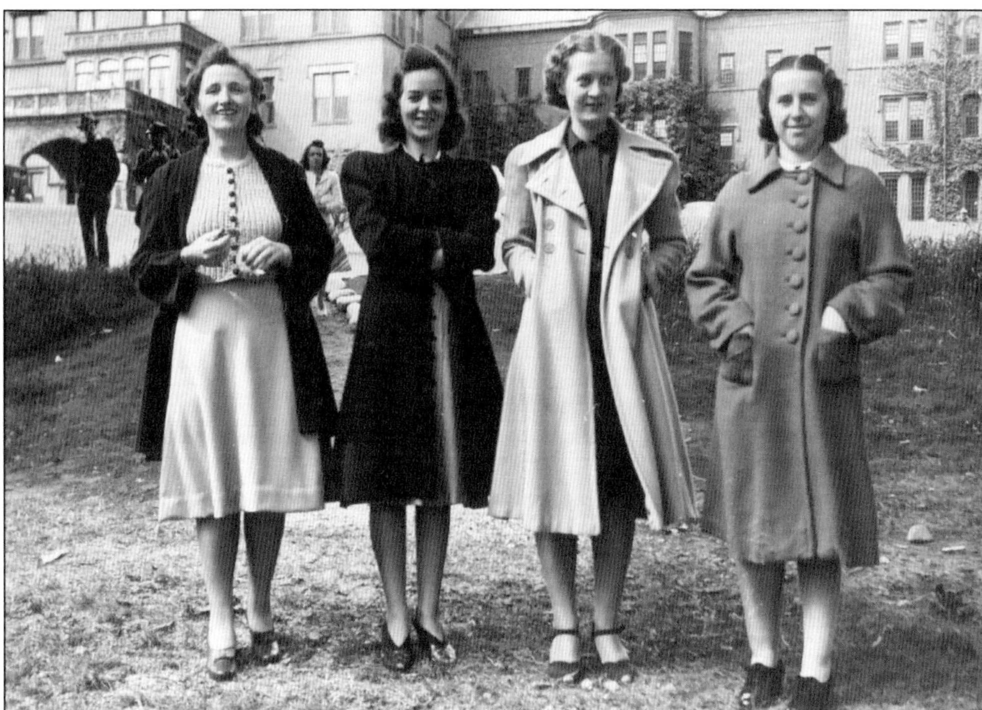

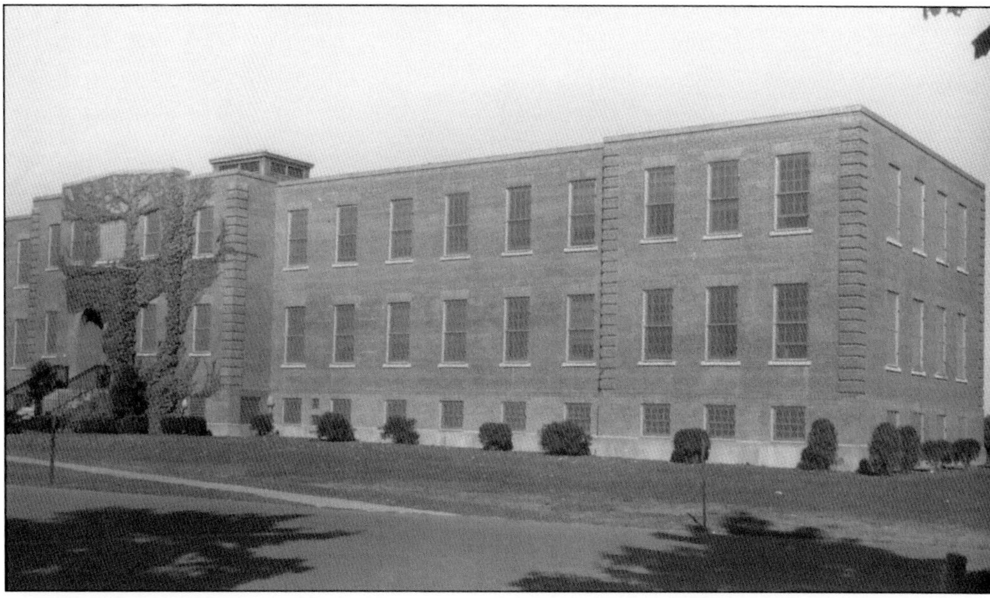

This structure opened in 1952 for the care of tubercular patients, who, until this time, were housed in overcrowded dormitories in the infirmary buildings. Six years later, it was converted to a general infirmary when tubercular patients were transferred to other hospitals. A freestanding structure when it was built, it was physically united into the Memorial Building complex with the construction of the G Building in 1969. It was named for deceased staffer Arthur Pruzynski, below left, who quit work as an attendant to enlist in the Army during World War II and died in combat in Germany. He stands with Dominic Mazilli in the courtyard behind Lower North 3 in the summer of 1937.

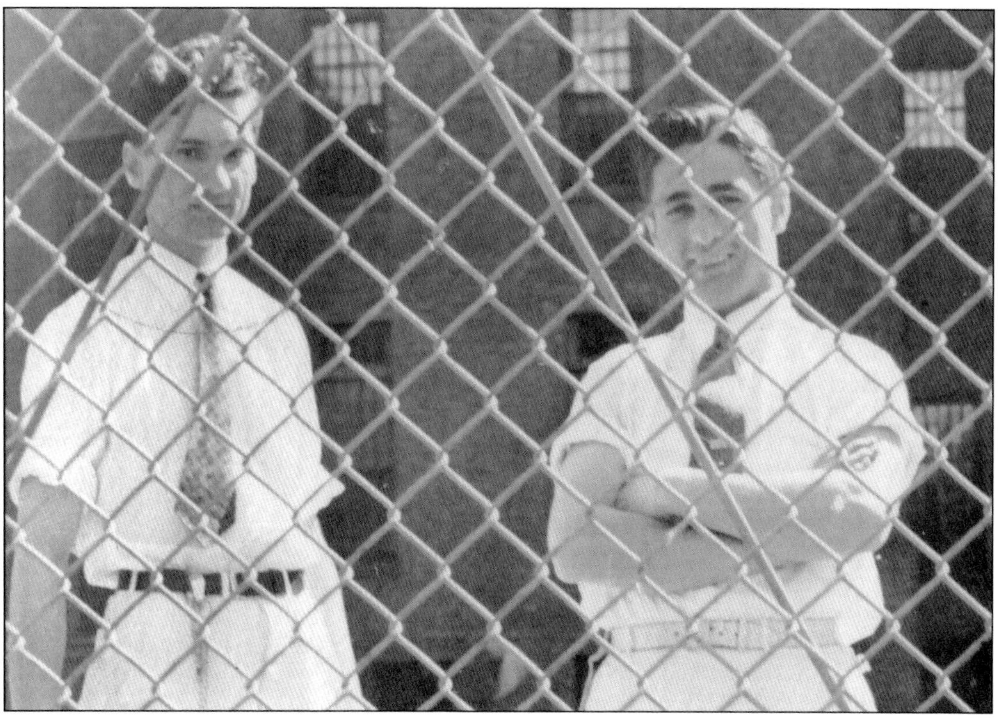

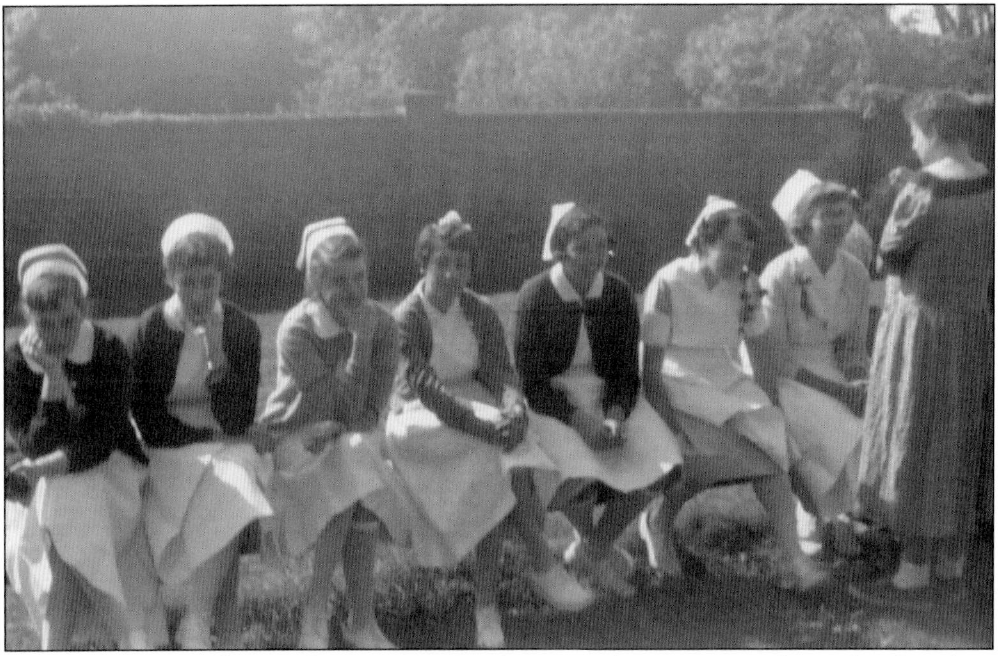

Nurses, on their graduation day, are enjoying the sun with a patient in the enclosed yard on the south side of the hospital. Patients' yards, "two for each sex, of a large size, with brick walks, shade trees," were intended to enable "many patients who wish to avoid the greater publicity of the grounds, to have the benefit of the open air," prescribed Thomas Kirkbride.

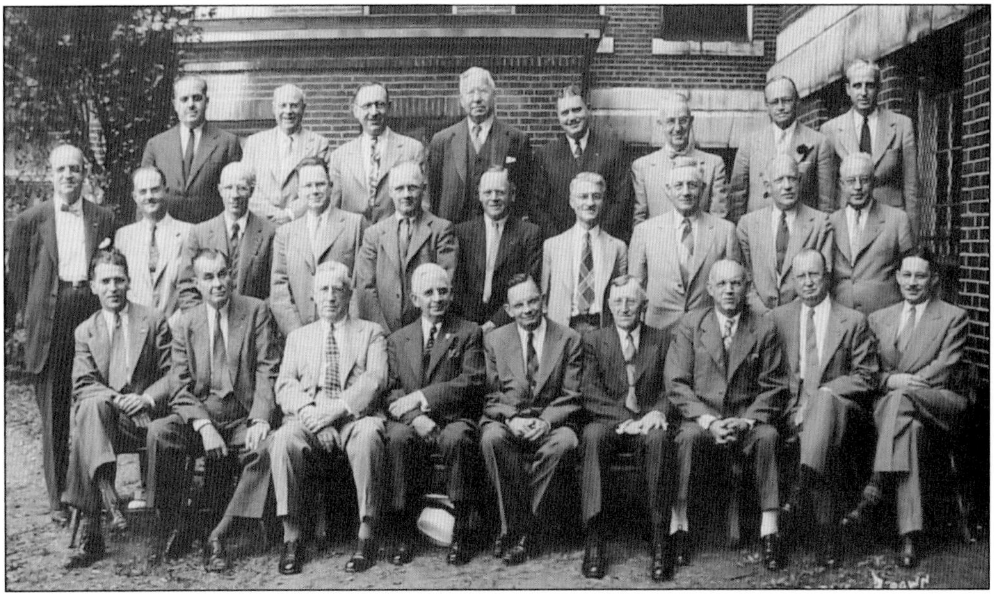

The mental health leaders of Massachusetts gather in 1945, almost exactly 100 years after the founding of the Association of Medical Superintendents of American Institutions for the Insane by the "original thirteen." Hospitals had proliferated across the country and now housed 462,000 patients nationwide. While occasional exposes brought the hospitals to public attention, most were out of sight and out of mind. But this 100-year-old system was in serious crisis, and change was brewing.

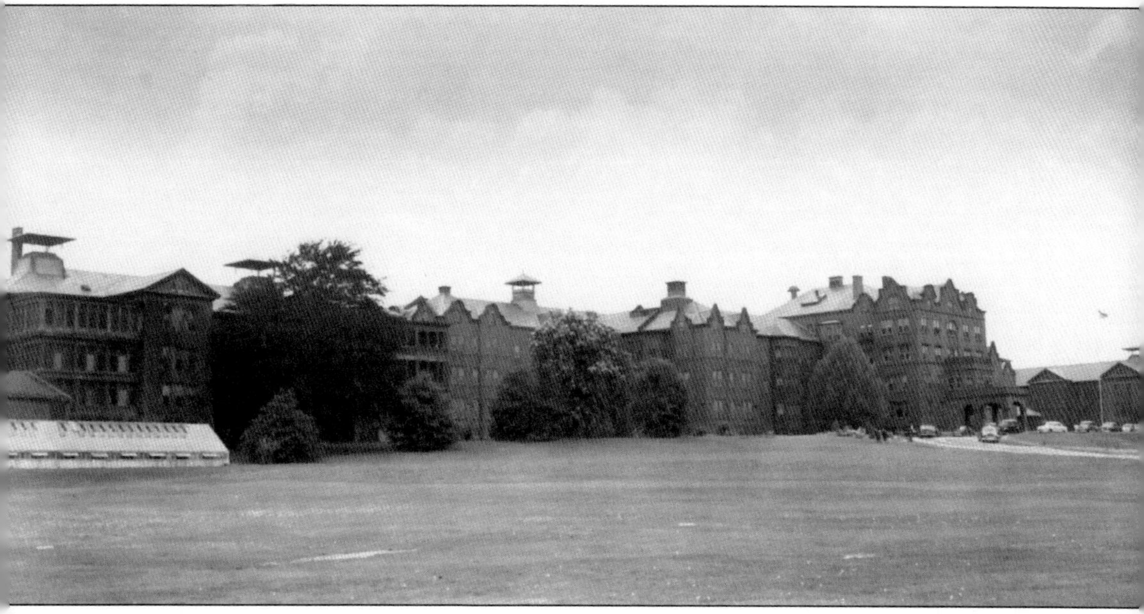

This view of the main buildings offers no clue to what was going on inside in 1952. In its 30 wards (and in a dozen more across the road in the Memorial Building complex), 2,384 souls were housed in rooms designed for 1,780. Newly admitted patients were brought to wards in the infirmaries to the left and right ends of the complex. These wards mixed new admissions with frail patients, those on suicide watch, and those undergoing electroconvulsive and insulin shock treatment. Severely disturbed male patients, whether their symptoms were acute or chronic, were housed together on one large ward holding 68 patients that extended across two halls in the rear of the north side. Several seclusion rooms were used there, but physical restraints were preferred because there were too few staff members to properly monitor everyone. In the comparable unit for females on the south side rear, the 10 seclusion rooms had no working lights and there were two toilets for 44 patients. These patients ate on the ward from trays on their laps because there were no tables for their use.

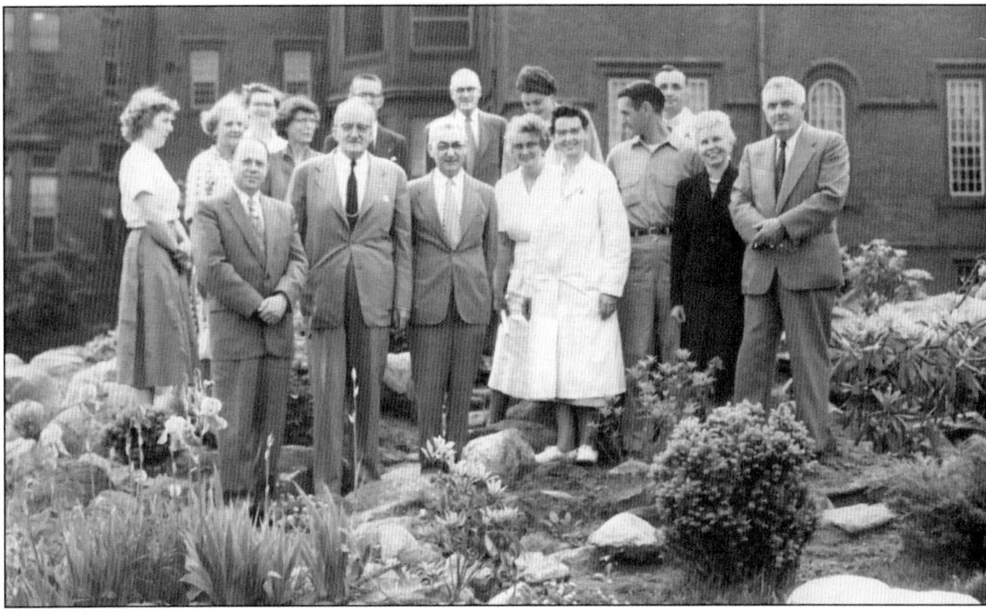

On the cusp of enormous change, when the hospital was at its largest and about to enter a period of dramatic decline in the number of patients, its leaders were gathered in the rock garden for this group portrait. Appearing on the occasion of the hospital's 100th birthday are, from left to right, (first row) Dr. Henry Benjamin; Dr. Fernand Longpre, superintendent; Dr. Philip Freedman; Mildred Bolton, head of housekeeping, and Florence "Sue" Eaton, director of nurses.

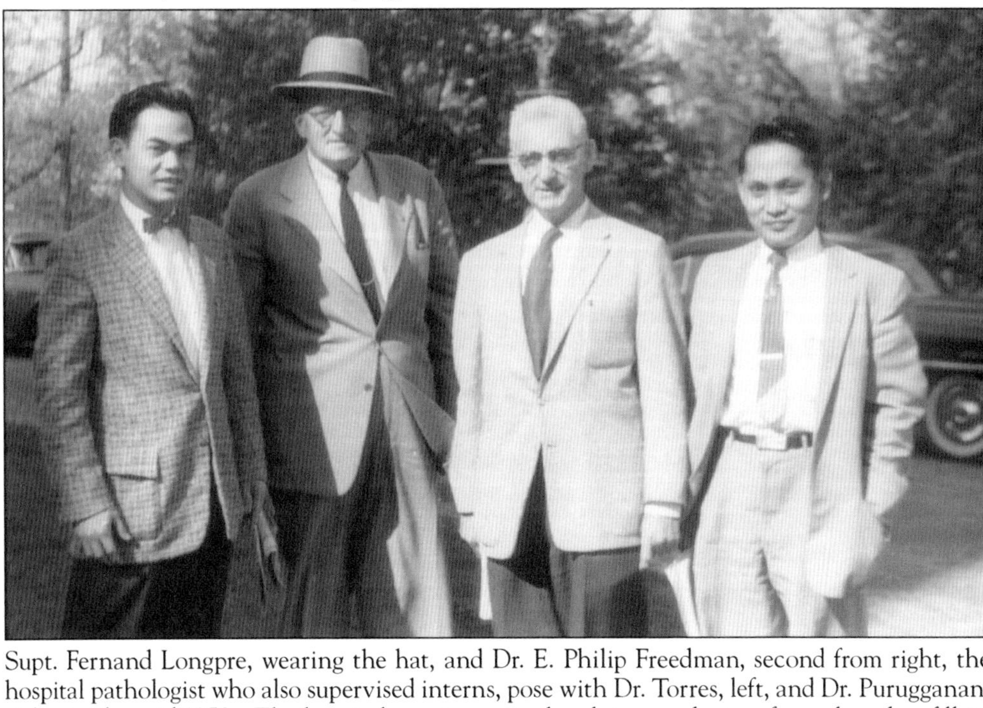

Supt. Fernand Longpre, wearing the hat, and Dr. E. Philip Freedman, second from right, the hospital pathologist who also supervised interns, pose with Dr. Torres, left, and Dr. Purugganan, right, in the mid-1950s. The hospital was increasingly relying on doctors from abroad to fill its medical positions. It was often noted that patients found it hard to communicate with doctors without good English language skills.

Three

CHANGE

Northampton State Hospital changed dramatically in the second half of the 20th century. It was forced by circumstance and public pressure to confront its shortcomings. It was challenged by a new activism from the national government, new advances in psychiatric treatment, new leaders not wed to the old ways, and committed activists determined to strike at the heart of an institution they saw as fundamentally flawed.

In the two decades after World War II, a new consensus developed in favor of mental health treatment in the community. While this goal differed from the hospital's founders, it was based on the same optimism about society's ability to cure mental illness. A newly powerful federal government became, for the first time, an instrument of policy reform in the field, redirecting resources to community treatment. The Medicare program opened a door through which hundreds of elderly patients walked out of the hospital.

New therapies were developed, most markedly in new drugs for the treatment of severe illness. This kindled new hope for assisting the chronically ill, lighting a fire under those who had been content to live with less. More trained psychiatric workers entered the field and coordinated treatment programs began to consider the whole environment of the patient as part of the therapy. In a sense, it was a renewal of the old notion of moral therapy. At Northampton, these changes were led by Supt. Harry Goodman and director of nurses Florence "Sue" Eaton, who put an end to business as usual.

Just as important, in the changed political climate of the 1960s, social and legal activists committed themselves to the cause of improving the life of those with mental illness and securing their civil and legal rights. Family members came out of the shadows to demand improvements, monitor conditions, and ultimately, to oversee and advise the entire system. Attorney Steven J. Schwartz led a legal challenge in the 1970s and 1980s that helped establish the most comprehensive community care system in America. In the process, the number of patients at the hospital would shrink from several thousand to a few dozen.

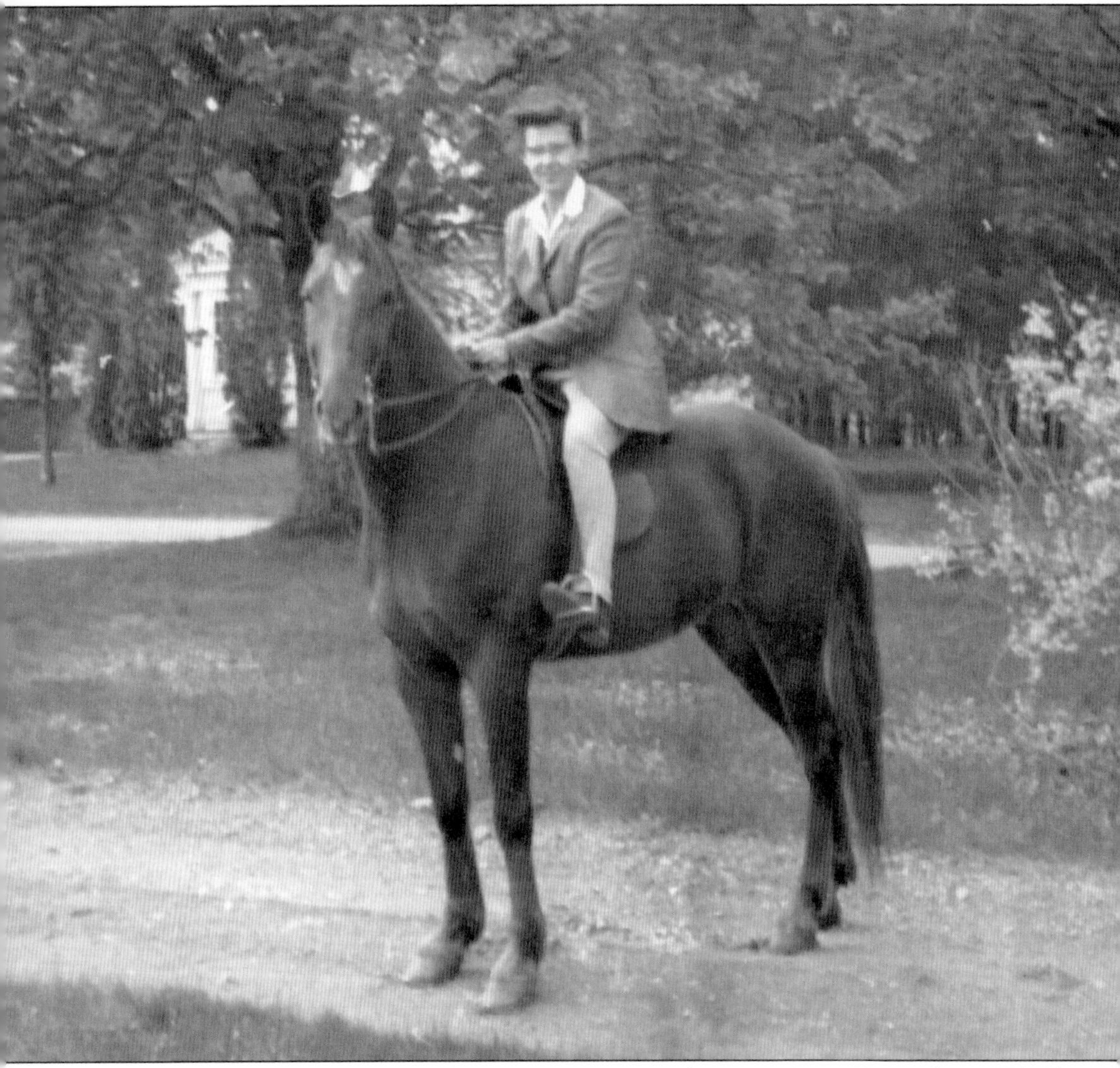

Florence "Sue" Eaton, director of nurses, came to Northampton State Hospital in 1953. She had a vision for improving the care of the patients and the toughness and tenacity to make changes in a stubbornly resistant institution. She was known for riding her Morgan horse around the grounds. One of her colleagues remembers Eaton's bold closing of a dank basement ward, which she found unacceptable for the patients, by nailing a board across the door, which read, "CONDEMNED!" Together with Superintendent Goodman, Eaton was able to usher in a new era at the hospital.

From left to right, Katherine "Katy" Powers, Phyllis Thomas, and Judith Ferrini are seen shopping in downtown Northampton in this 1957 photograph. They are beginning their three-month course in psychiatric nurses training at the state hospital. Katy and Phyllis married brothers William and Donald Duffus who both worked at the hospital as attendants. Both women had long careers as nurses at Northampton State and played important roles in reducing the number of patients in the hospital in the 1970s and 1980s.

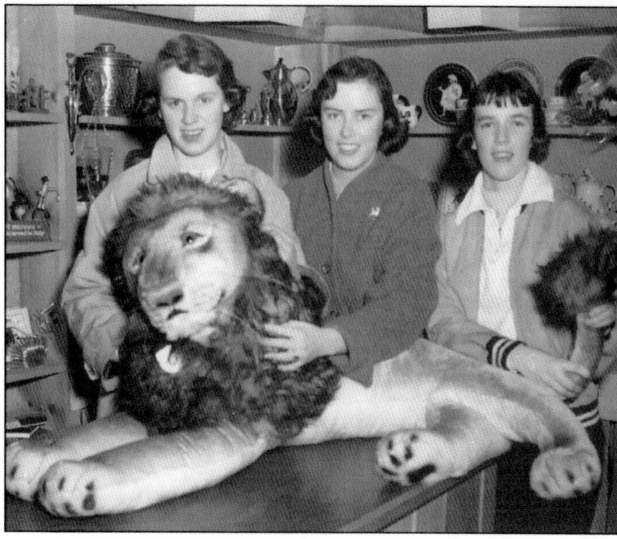

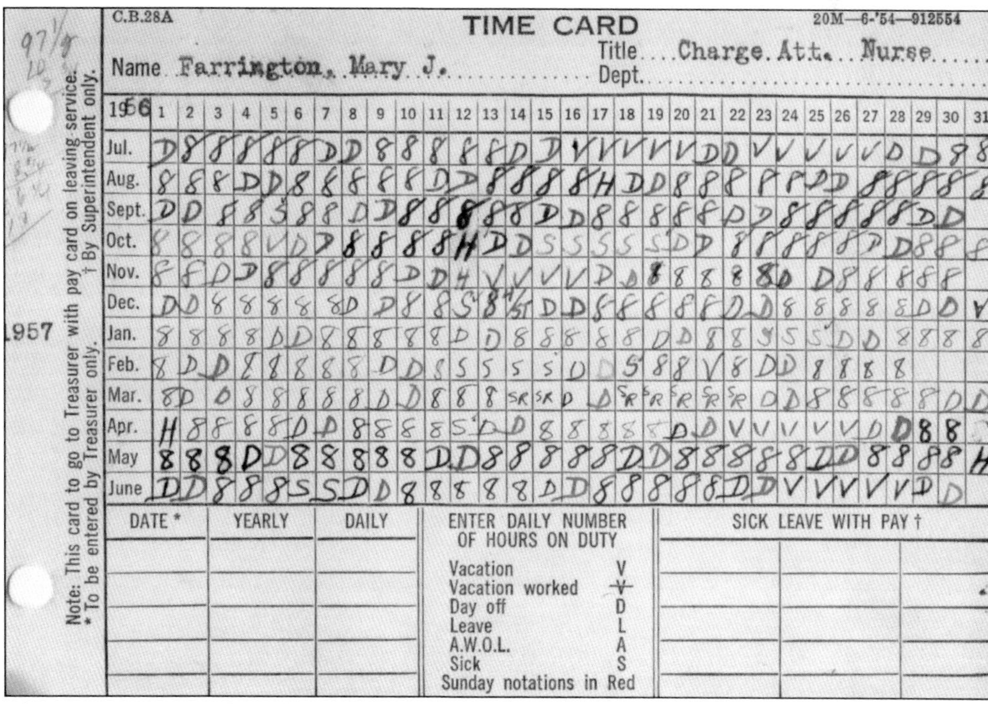

C.B.28A

TIME CARD

20M—6-'54—912554

Name Farrington, Mary J.

Title Charge. Att. Nurse

Dept.

1956 — Jul., Aug., Sept., Oct., Nov., Dec.; 1957 — Jan., Feb., Mar., Apr., May, June; days 1–31

Note: This card to go to Treasurer with pay card on leaving service.
* To be entered by Treasurer only. † By Superintendent only.

DATE *	YEARLY	DAILY	ENTER DAILY NUMBER OF HOURS ON DUTY	SICK LEAVE WITH PAY †

ENTER DAILY NUMBER OF HOURS ON DUTY
Vacation V
Vacation worked V̶
Day off D
Leave L
A.W.O.L. A
Sick S
Sunday notations in Red

This is a nurse's time sheet from 1956–1957. The employees at the hospital were deeply connected to the life of the institution. "We spent every day on these same floors. We lived with these patients five days a week, we became part of their family. I can't say that for every single floor, it's like any human service," remembers Nancy, a former employee. Another remembers being told during his orientation week, "When you leave work every day, leave the hospital underneath the front steps."

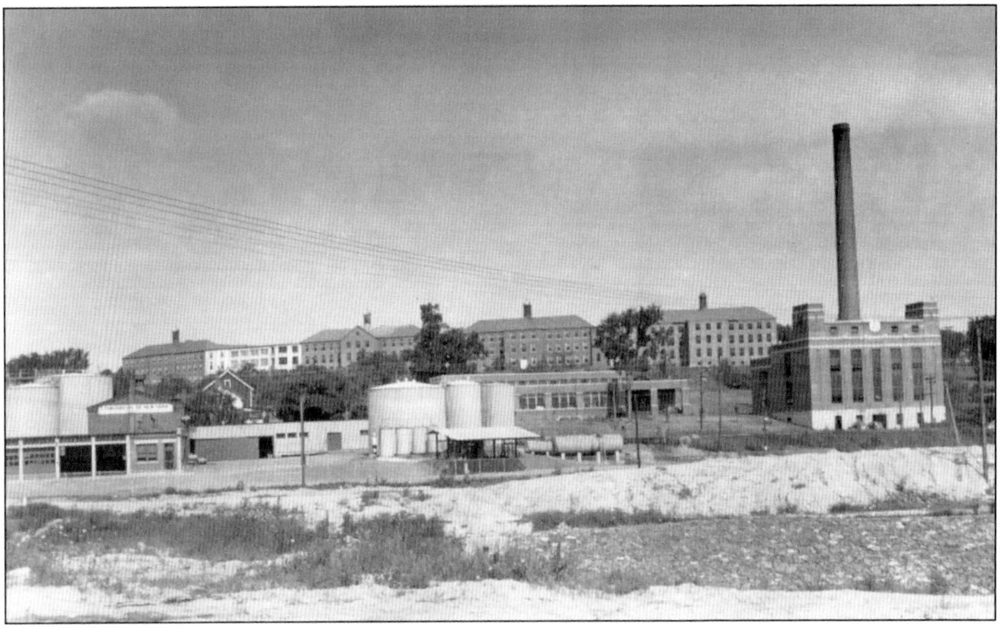

This view from Earle Street shows the Memorial Building complex on the hill. The attached wards, each with a cupola in the center, are the C, D, E, and F Buildings. Completed by 1936, these buildings were used to ease the overcrowding in the main buildings by transferring the long-term "chronic" patients there. In the middle ground are the low-slung laundry and the power plant with a chimney, both New Deal public works projects.

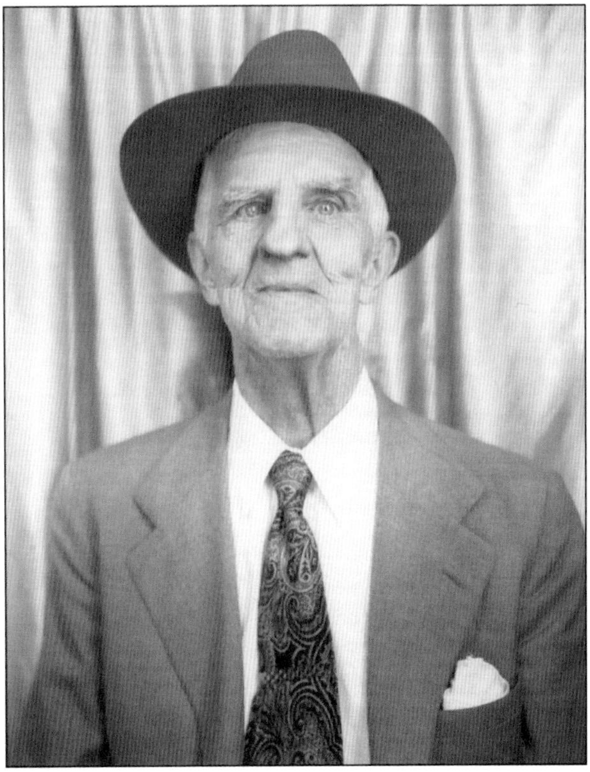

Isaac Heald was a patient resident at the hospital for decades. He was widely known as a friendly and gentle person, who always dressed up and always tipped his hat in greeting. He lived on a parole ward and walked downtown on his own. He had sufficient money, and when asked by the staff why he stayed on at the hospital replied, "This is my home. I'm not leaving." The photograph is from 1955.

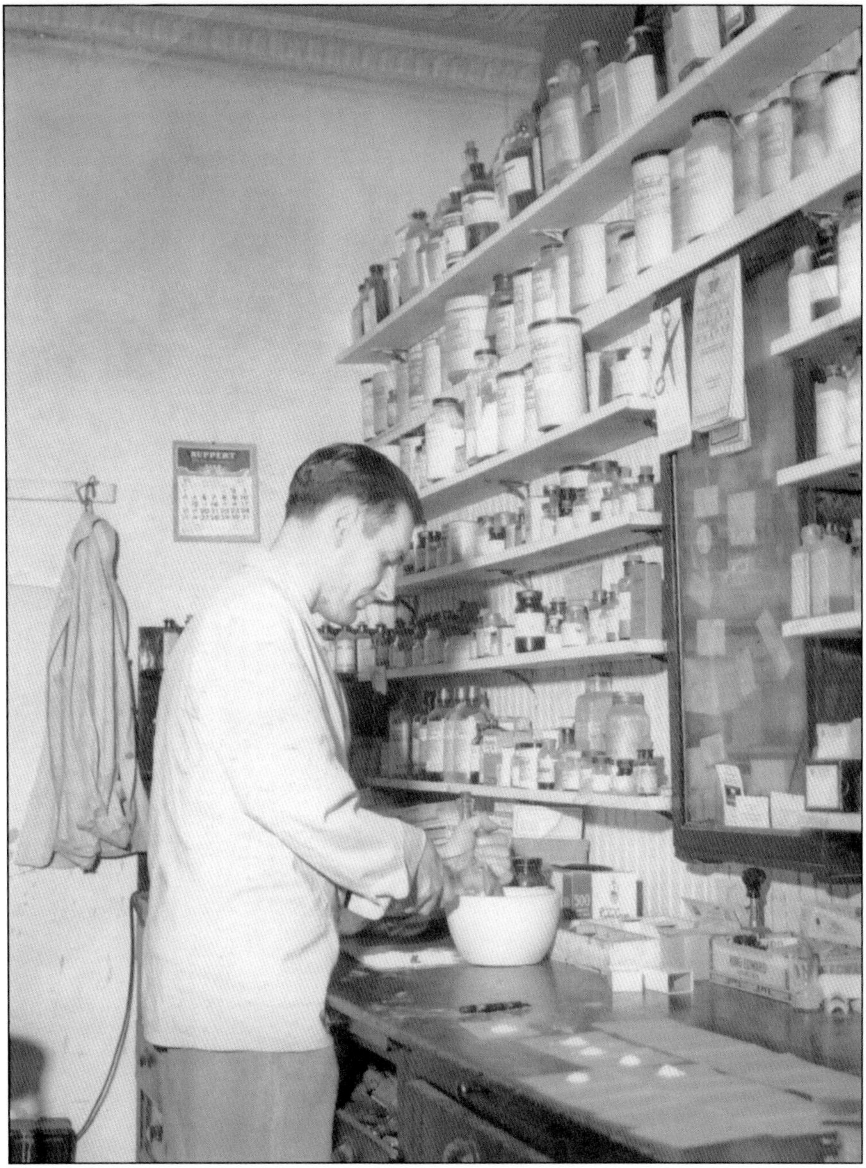

A variety of medications were administered to patients from the earliest days of the state hospitals. But it was only in the 1950s with the development of powerful tranquilizers and effective antidepressants that drugs became a key component of treatment. Thorazine and Serpasil were first used at the hospital in 1954 with a few "chronically disturbed" patients. Two years later the superintendent observed "quieter and cleaner" geriatric wards with less resort to seclusion and restraint, as the drugs seemed effective in managing anxiety, agitation, and manic states. Acutely ill patients were treated with the same drugs, leading to a large reduction in the use of electric shock therapy. In 1956, the new anti-tranquilizing drug Marsilid was introduced, offering some hope for improvement in the large number of "chronically regressed and withdrawn" patients. A flood of new drugs was introduced in the next decades. The explosion in drug therapy, while contributing to a new optimism, also created new problems with serious side effects and long-term risk to those using them. Shown is Frank Sullivan, the hospital pharmacist, mixing preparations in the pharmacy, where he served from 1942 until 1976.

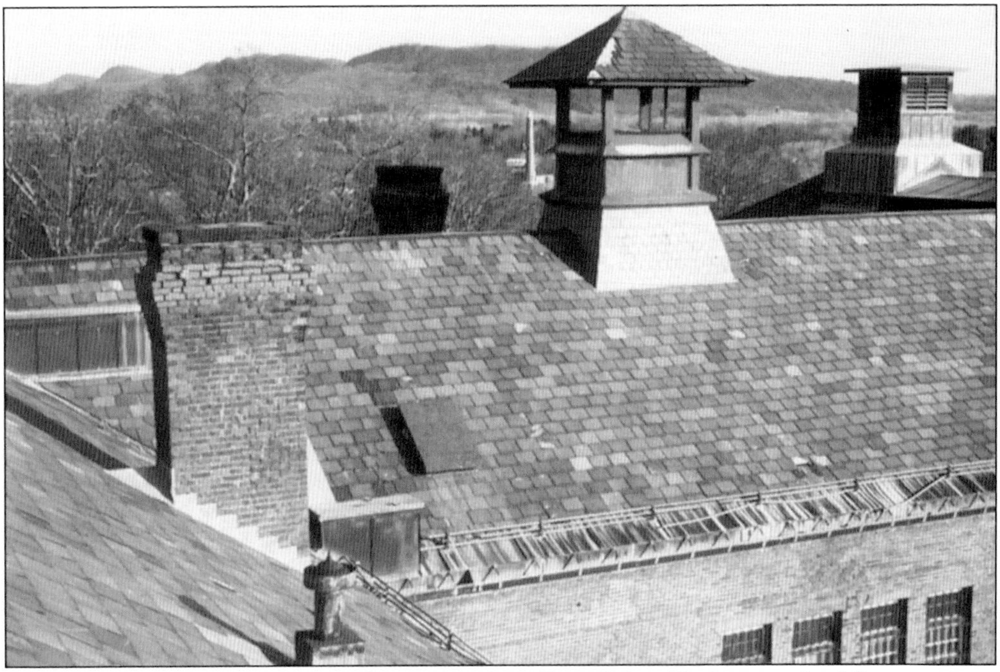

In a 1952 letter, while she was a student at Smith College, Sylvia Plath wrote the following about seeing Northampton State Hospital: "We changed then, for the cocktail party, and walked over to the professor's house. On the way we decided to keep on walking for a while longer, and so we walked up to the mental hospital, among the buildings, listening to the people screaming. It was a most terrifying, holy experience, with the sun setting red and cold over the black hills, and the inhuman, echoing howls coming from the barred windows."

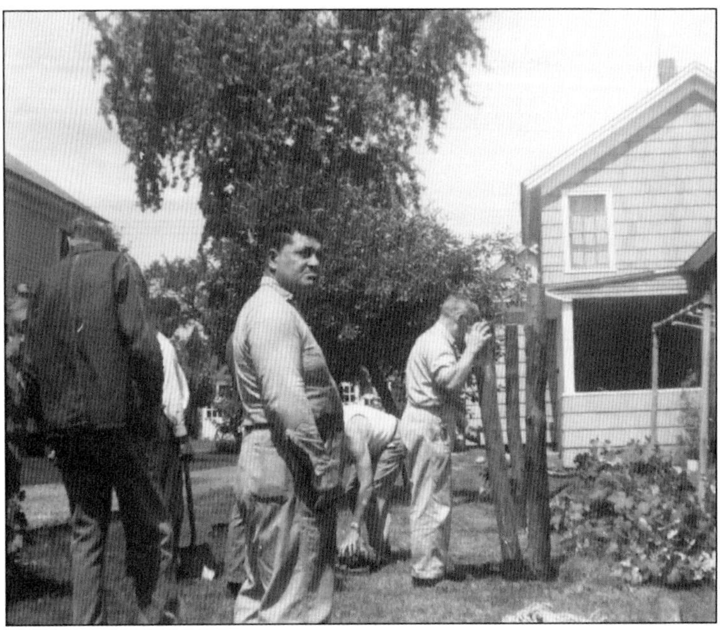

Some patients worked for families in the neighborhood of the hospital since at least the 1920s. They helped with housework and even cared for children. Claude Hill, on the right, leads a group of unidentified patients in a project to beautify the garden of his home. For many years, Hill supervised a work crew of patients whose job it was to scour and clean the network of tunnels that connected the primary buildings of the hospital.

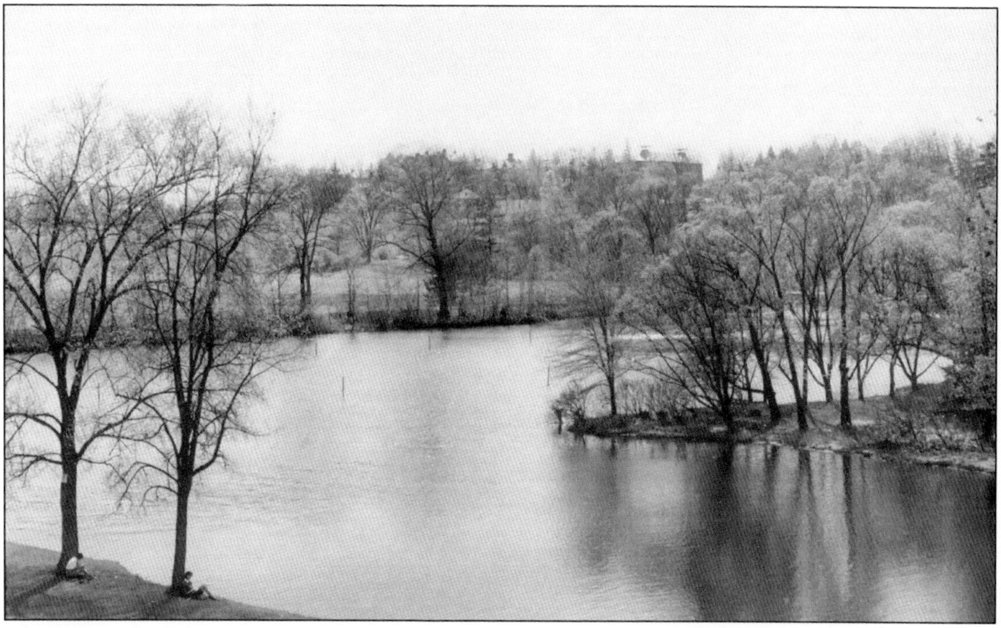

The hospital was a constant presence in the city of Northampton, not only because so many local residents worked at the hospital, but also because its location directly across the hill from Smith College was so prominent. Smith College and the hospital shared Paradise Pond between them, which blurred the edges of the two institutions. When the sun went down, the hospital could be seen from the Smith College campus, clearly silhouetted against the sky.

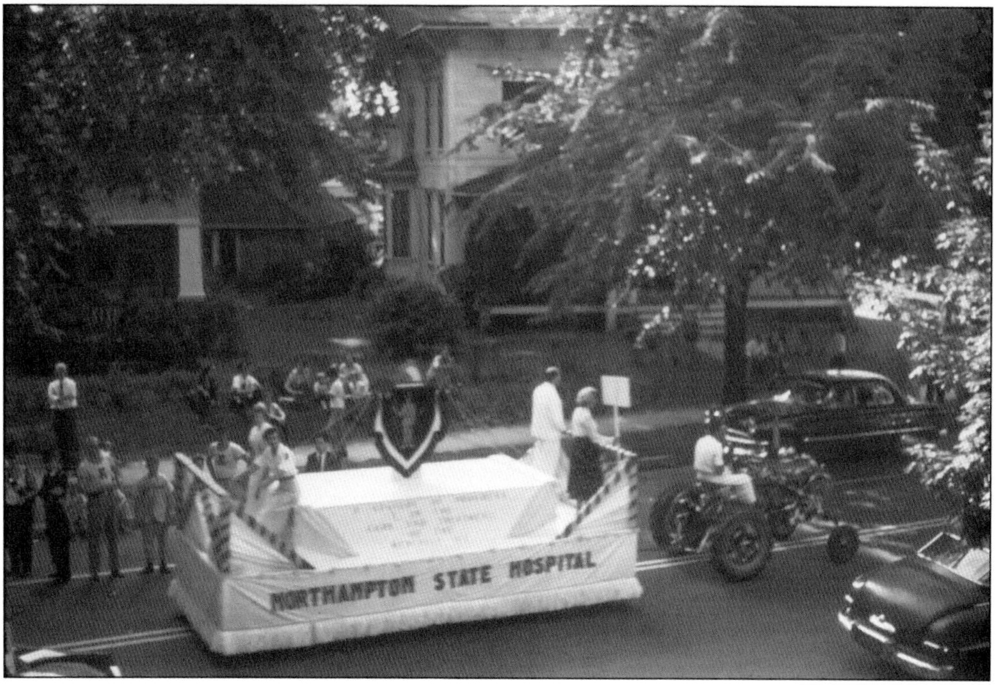

The occupational therapy staff members ride the state hospital float at the rear of the Northampton Tercentennial Parade in 1954, celebrating "a century of progress in the care of the mentally ill."

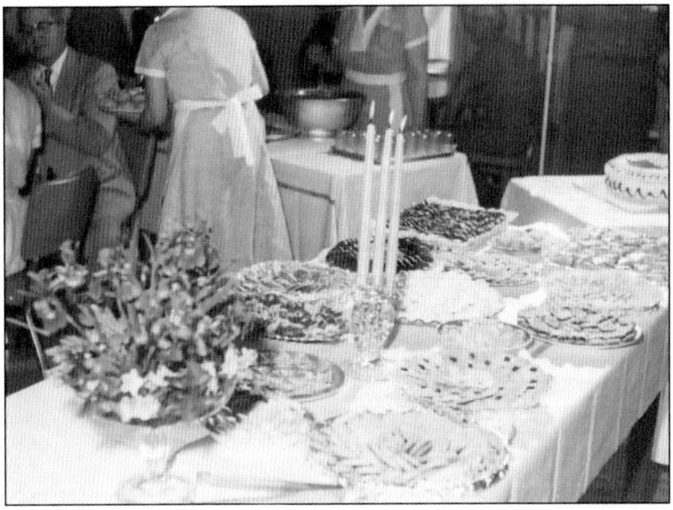

At a time when the hospital prepared and served 8,000 meals each day, the hospital staff also prepared this opulent spread in 1959 for the retirement party of Frank Smith. Smith, appointed steward in 1919, described his role as supervising the purchase and serving of food, as well as writing the specifications for purchasing, installing, and maintaining all buildings and equipment. Dr. Harry Goodman, superintendent, is seated in the upper left.

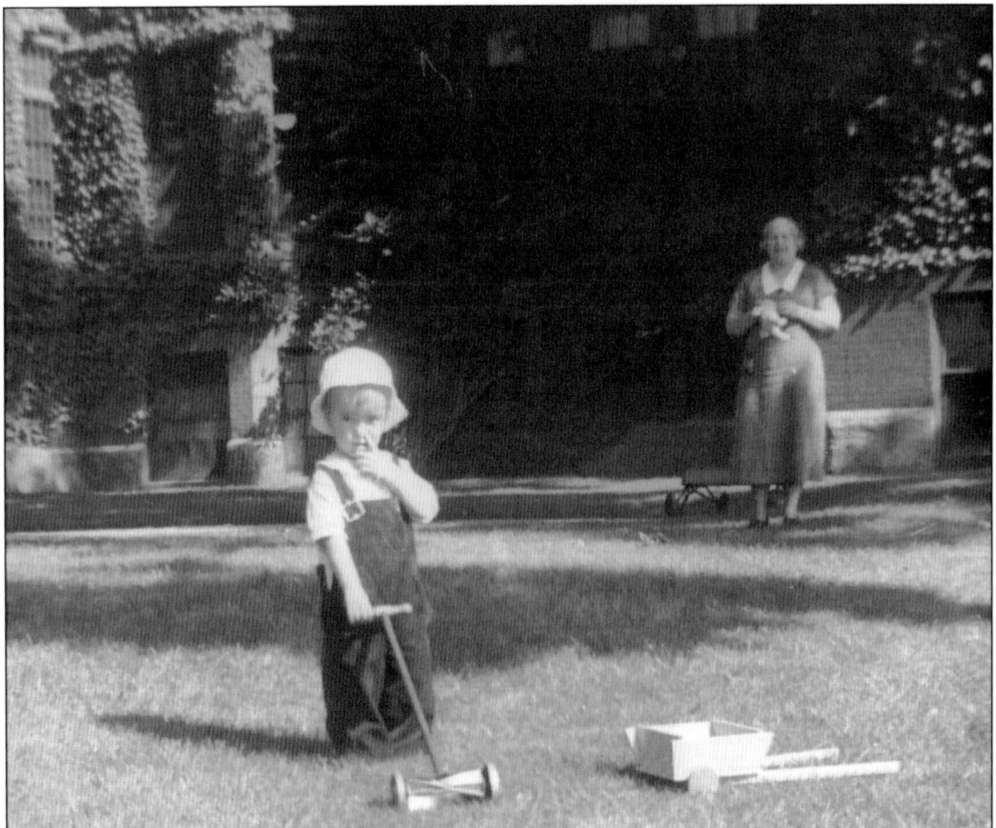

Many children grew up in the shadow of the hospital. Some were the children of doctors who lived on the grounds, and others were the children of workers who lived in the nearby neighborhood. One remembered her childhood: "We bowled over there and played around the grounds. They used to have entertainment for the patients and we could go. We grew up with them and accepted them as another person, same as your neighbors." The woman and child are unidentified.

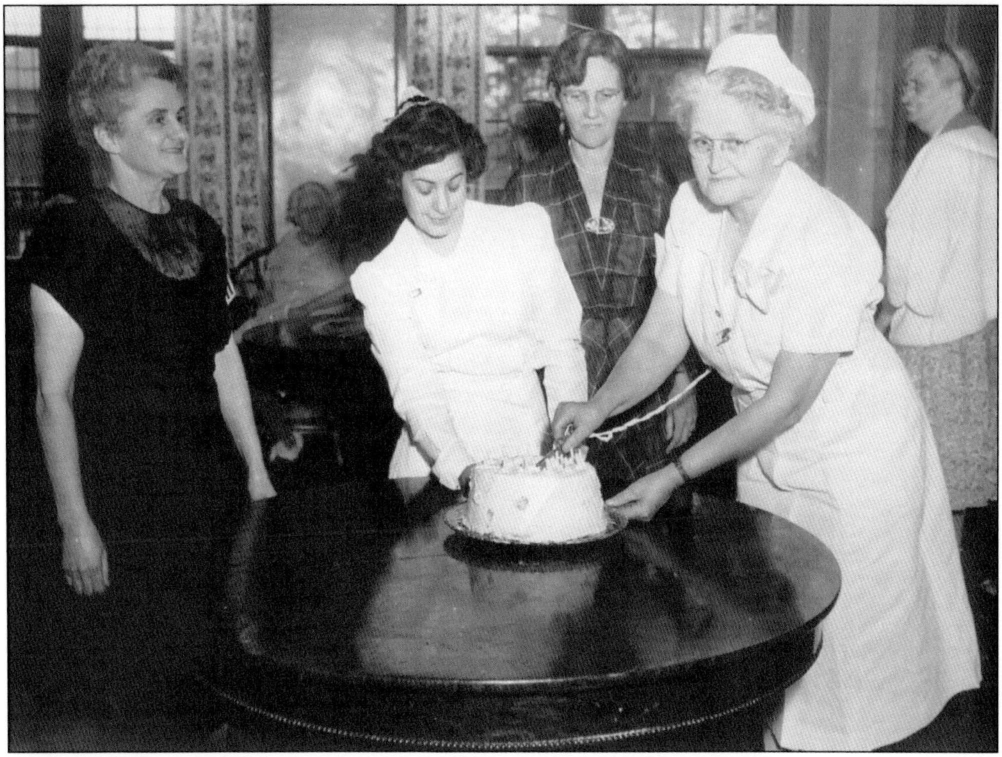

This is a scene from life on a ward in the 1950s. With Mrs. Federal Bridgman looking on, nurse Ashley Stevens appears to cut a cake with her keys, perhaps because knives were not allowed on the ward. Another employee looks back at that time as follows: "I remember them bringing in a girl from Pittsfield, she had this infatuation with Eddie Fisher, the singer. Believe it or not, they brought her to the state hospital for that. And I remember the doctor saying to the parents, 'Don't visit, because the less you visit the quicker she is going to get used to the place.' That's what they used to tell the families. Very few people came in with families, very few. It was mostly police who brought them in."

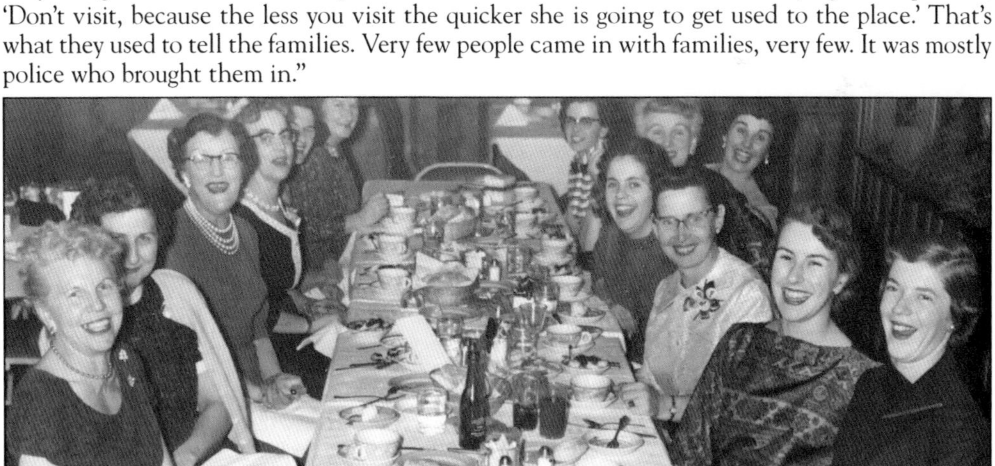

At a Christmas celebration in 1955, the hospital office staff joins director of nurses Florence "Sue" Eaton. Seated on the left side of the table are, from left to right, Vera Frennier, Myrtle Kuczynski, Sally Gulow, Ruth Stearns, Sue Arel Plath, and Marion Barton. Seated on the right side are, from left to right, Yolande Korona, Gloria Borowski, Helen Blanchard, Meg Kearn, Eaton, Gail Landry, and Sue Harlow.

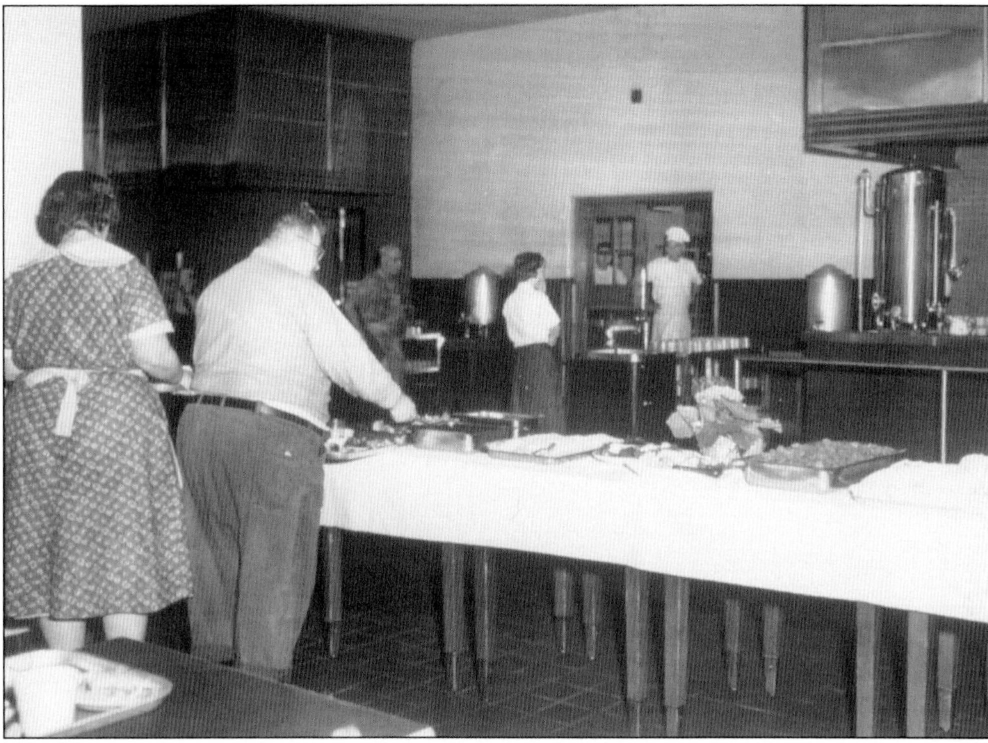

"The entire ward would take their trip through the tunnels to the main dining area. There were a lot of people eating at once. It almost seemed the entire state hospital would eat there at once. Does anyone remember the hot pastrami sandwiches we ate on Wednesday? Today there's nothing special about hot pastrami sandwiches, but they were something. They were so good that I would look over everyone else's tray, just to see if they finished theirs. They must have been good because everyone ate them down," said a former patient in 2000.

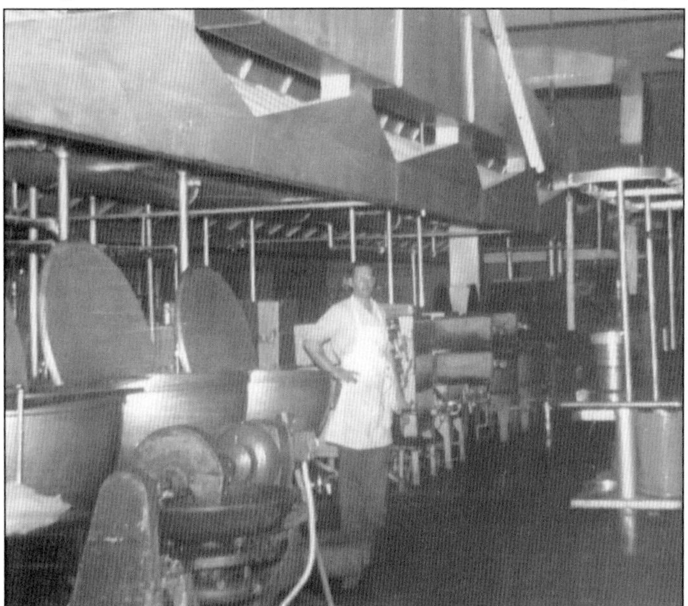

A new kitchen and dining room were completed in 1938, serving the entire hospital. Prior to this, patients in the main building were being served in 25 different dining rooms, all overcrowded and many flowing into day space. The kitchen space was so inadequate that "it [was] necessary to begin frying fish 3 hours before it [was] served to the patients," the hospital trustees reported in 1935. The new addition included a cannery, a bakery, vegetable preparation room, and a pathological lab.

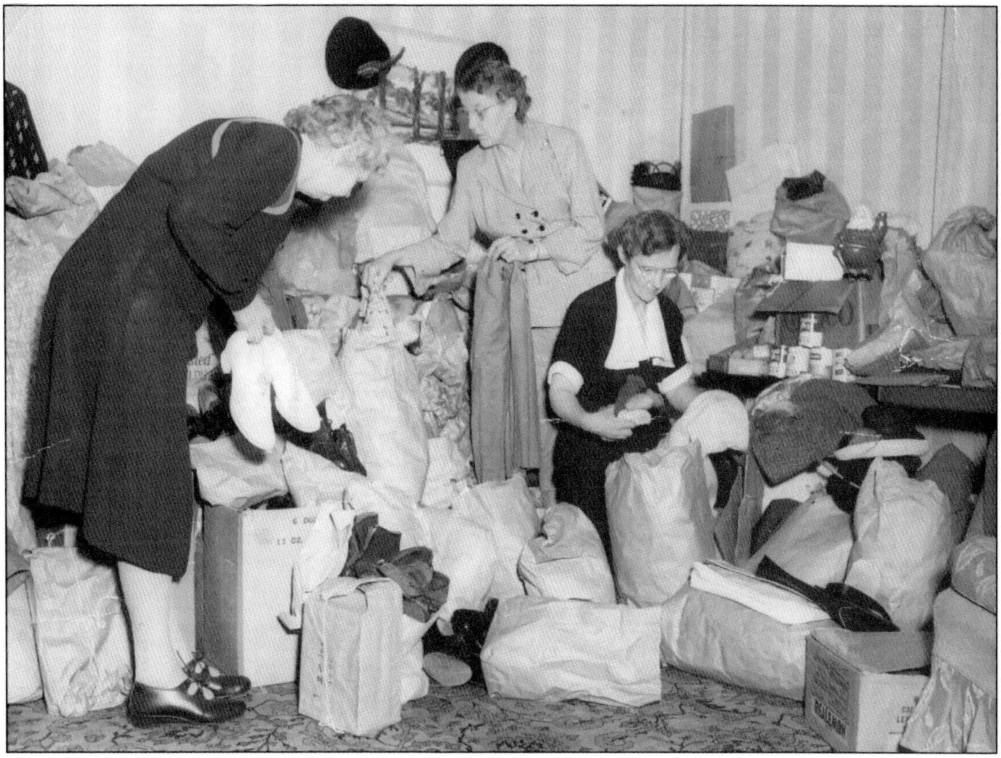

Members of Hilltop Friends, a volunteer organization, are sorting through their first collection of donated clothing in May 1950. This was an important and useful undertaking. The hospital housed 2,000 mostly long-term patients, many with little or no contact with friends or family. The making, marking, and cleaning of clothes for the patients required significant effort. Having clean, noninstitutional clothing was highly desirable. Kneeling is Mrs. Federal Bridgman.

A gift of new nightclothes for female patients is presented by a delegation of women representing the Holyoke Council of Churches to two grateful nurses. Leaders of the Hilltop Friends flank them. In the 1950s, the hospital, under the influence of Florence "Sue" Eaton, made sustained efforts to involve more people from the community in the life of the hospital.

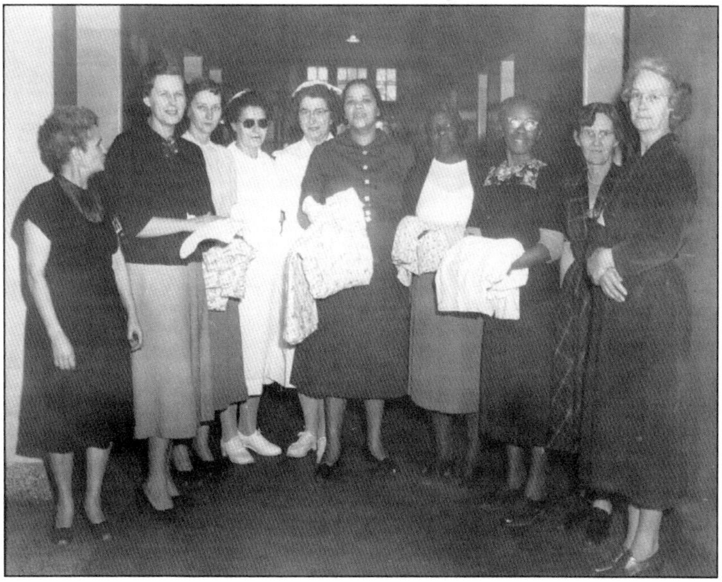

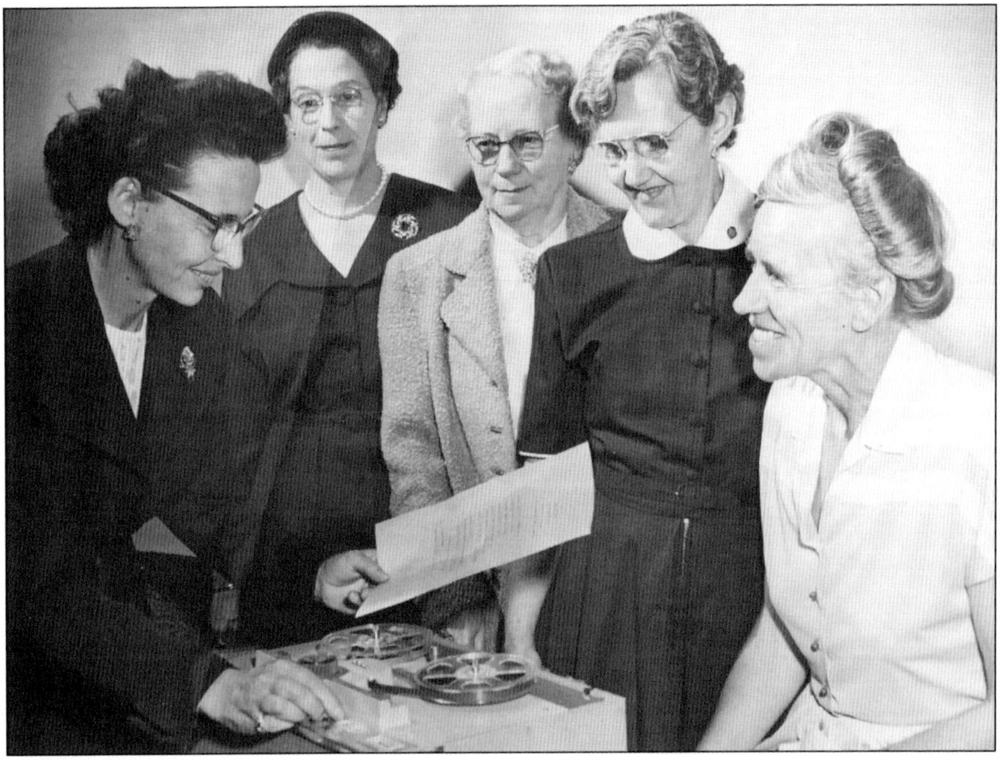

A tape recorder was donated to the hospital by leaders of the Hilltop Friends at their sixth annual meeting in 1956. Sue Eaton accepts the gift from, from left to right, Dorothy Stoddard of South Hadley, Eva Pall of Holyoke, Mrs. Federal Bridgman of Florence, and Marion Parsons of Southampton.

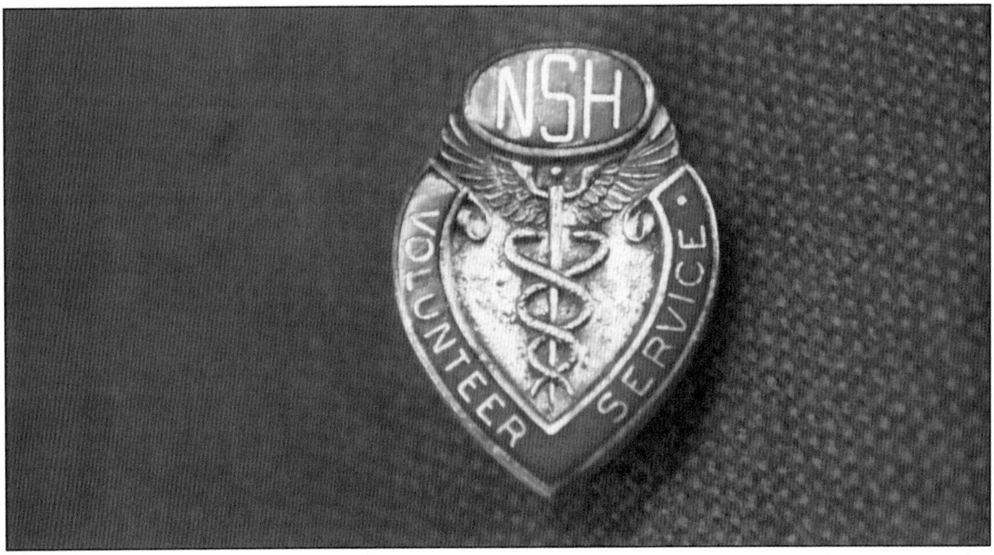

More than 40 civic groups, women's clubs, and church organizations were helping out at the hospital by the mid-1960s, as the hospital's efforts to involve the community bore fruit. 600 people were taking patients into their homes for visits, and the Nine College Volunteer Program won a national award for excellence.

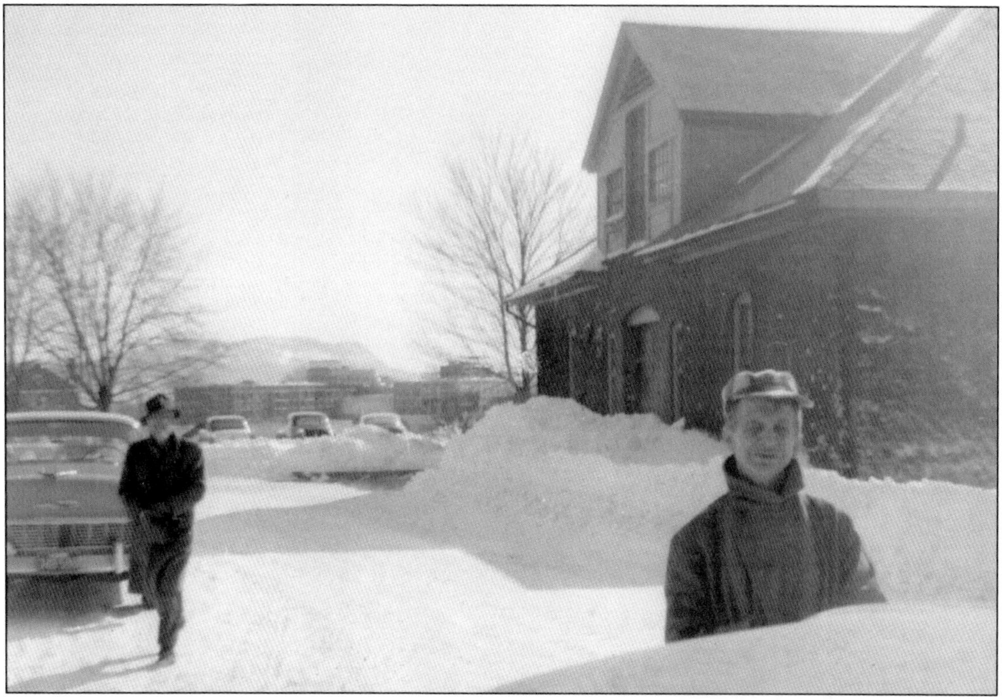

This winter scene was taken in the back of the hospital, near the carriage house, in 1958. The two men are unidentified. Those patients who had parole could move around the grounds freely, even go into town. One doctor remembers, "I think a more porous institution is a healthier one. A patient once escaped who bought a ticket to Hawaii. But he came back saying that it is better here than in the shelters of Honolulu. He thought he was going to be lying on the beach and pulling down coconuts. He called me from there, very cordial, and said, 'I'll be back soon!'"

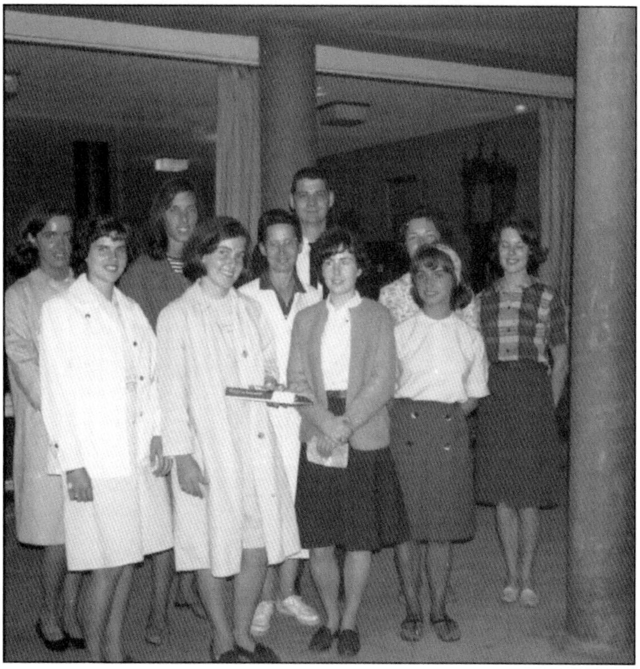

In the 1960s, hundreds of students from area colleges volunteered to spend time on the wards with patients one evening each week. They played board and card games or played music and led singing. In addition to the direct benefits to patients from having visitors, Sue Eaton, director of nurses, believed the program improved the standing of the hospital and the attitudes and commitment of the staff. Eaton poses here with volunteers from Mount Holyoke College.

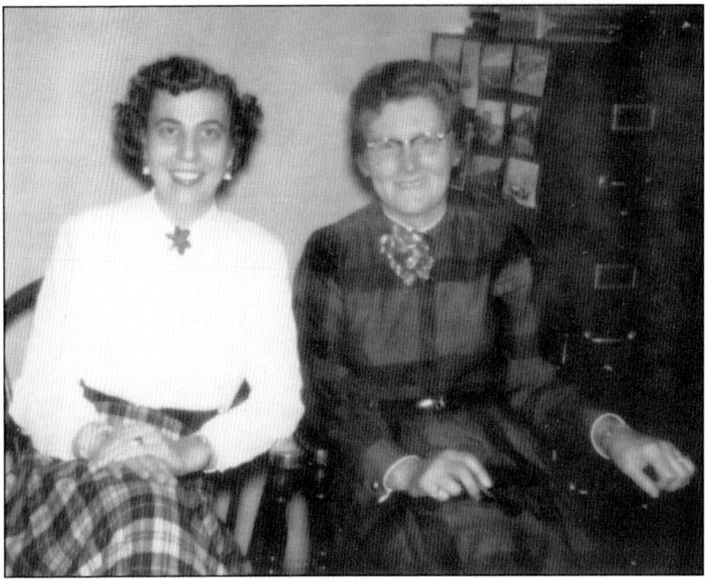

Massachusetts mandated the employment of female doctors at the state hospitals in 1884. Since that time, one and often several women doctors have been on the staff of the hospital. Dr. Shirley Gallup, left, was hired to staff the admissions ward in the new building that opened in 1959. Dr. Ruth Parker Haskell, right, had been on the staff since 1934, and after her death in 1961, the building was renamed in her honor.

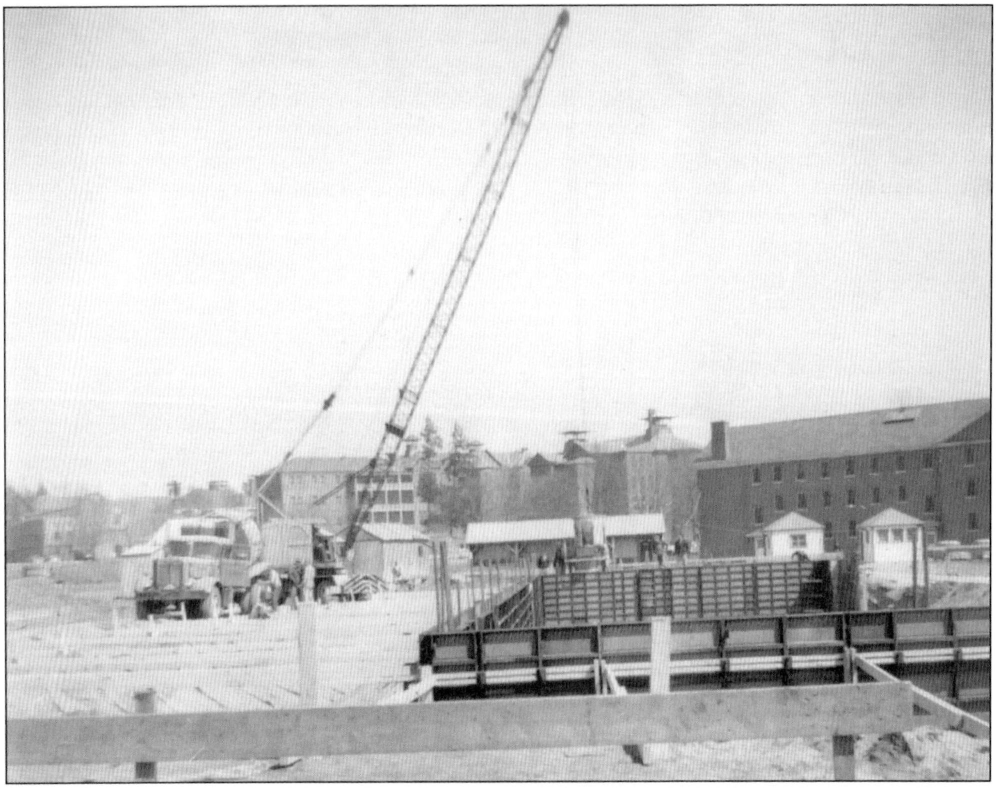

Construction of Haskell Building, the new admissions and intensive treatment structure, cost $2.5 million and was accompanied with much hope for pointing the hospital to a brighter, more medically oriented future. Designed as a three-story "acute treatment center" for 146 beds, it included a cafeteria, dayrooms, barbershop, beauty parlor, dental office, and occupational therapy suites. All around Massachusetts, state hospitals were being modernized with additions of such new buildings, made to resemble general hospitals.

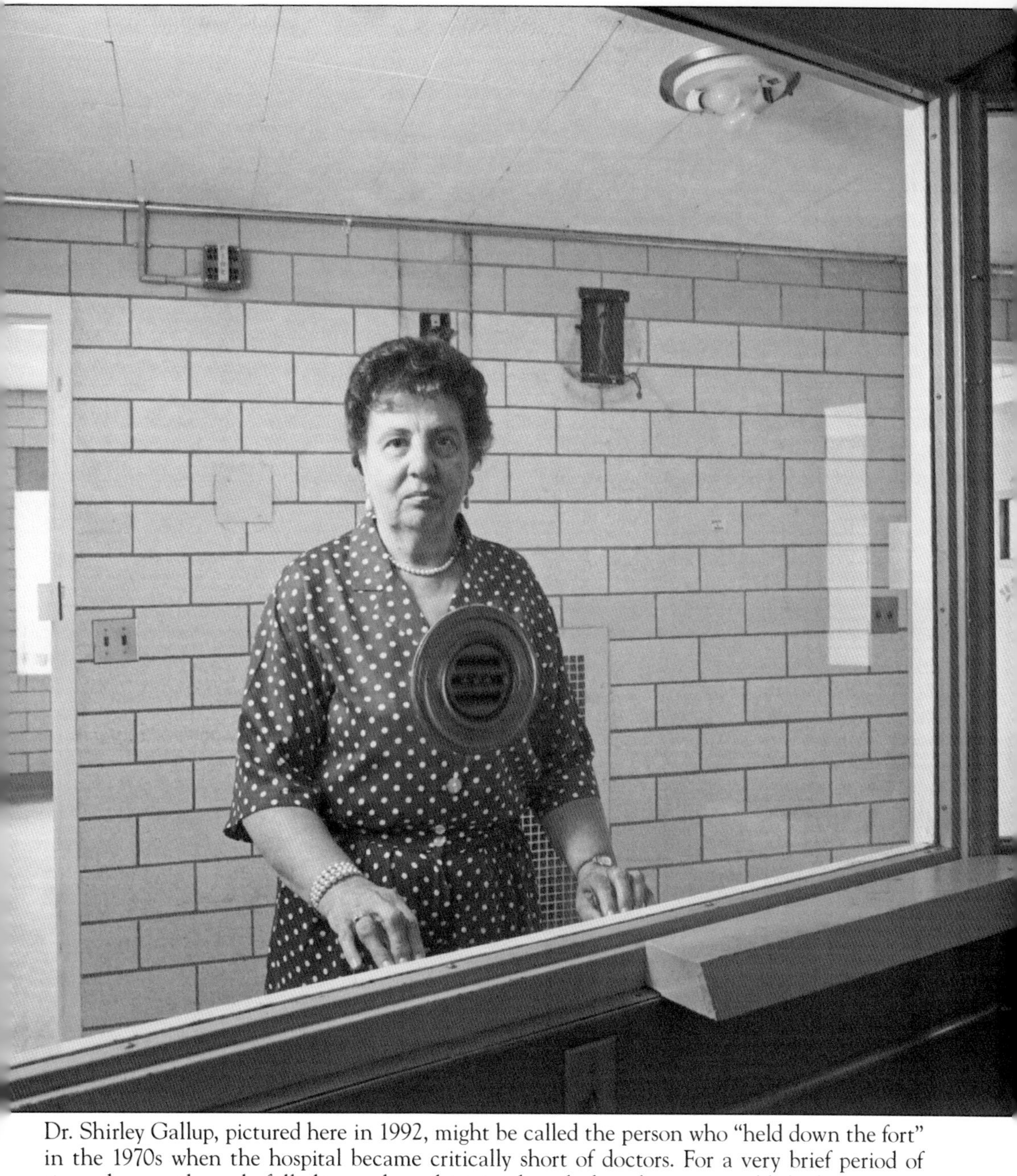

Dr. Shirley Gallup, pictured here in 1992, might be called the person who "held down the fort" in the 1970s when the hospital became critically short of doctors. For a very brief period of time, she was the only fully licensed psychiatrist there before the state established a contract for medical services with the University of Massachusetts Medical School. Only her deep commitment to the hospital and its patients kept her going through that period. She was hired to open the new admission ward in the Haskell Building and worked with the newly admitted patients there. Even though there was no time for individual psychotherapy, she organized group sessions. One such group with manic-depressive patients that began in 1964 continued to meet together socially with her nearly 30 years later, even though all had been long released from the hospital. (Courtesy of Stan Sherer.)

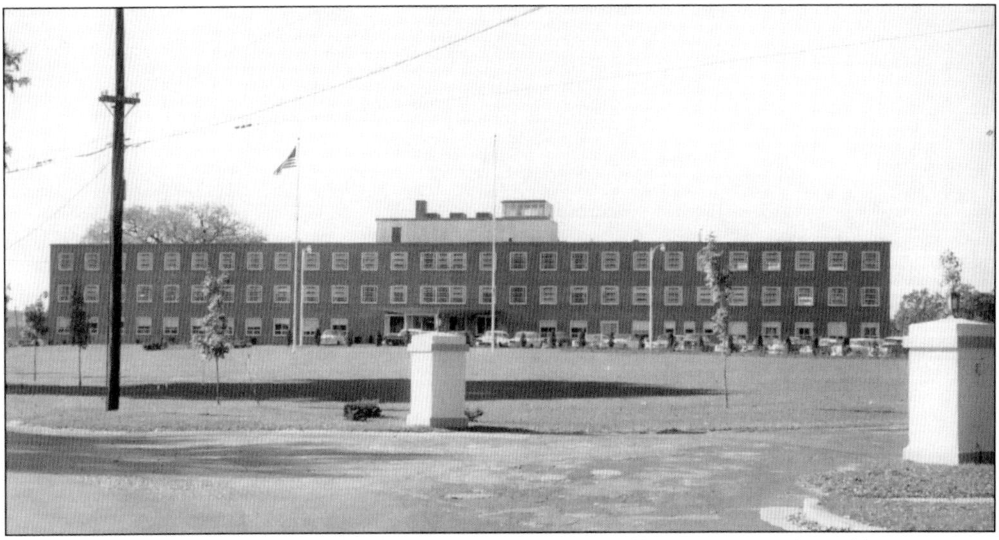

The Haskell Building opened in 1959 and became the most visible structure to the public passing on Route 66. It was the new focus of the life of Northampton State Hospital—intensive therapy. During the first year, it averaged 90 admissions per month. Today, it is the last remaining hospital building still in use, serving offices of the Department of Mental Health of Western Massachusetts.

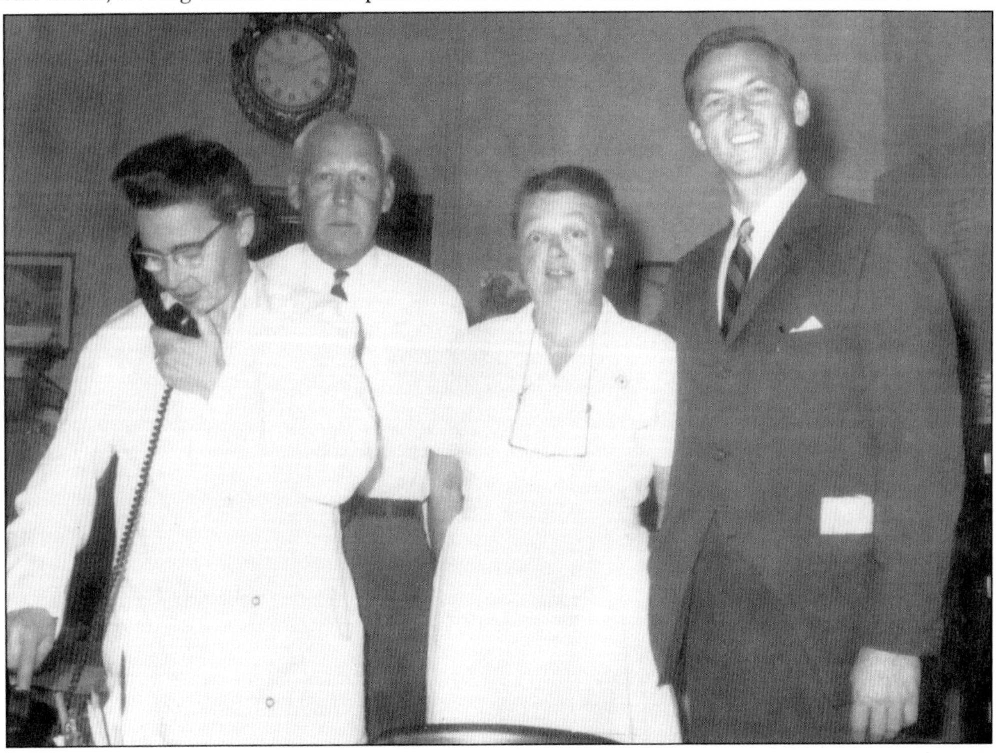

"It was quite customary for political hopefuls to arrive before elections to make the rounds with the superintendent and contact as many of us as they could," remembers one employee. Here, former governor Endicott Peabody, right, visits during his run for the US Senate in 1966. A Mr. Sampson and Peg Curran, chief nursing supervisor, seem unimpressed. Florence Eaton is on the telephone and seems too busy to be bothered.

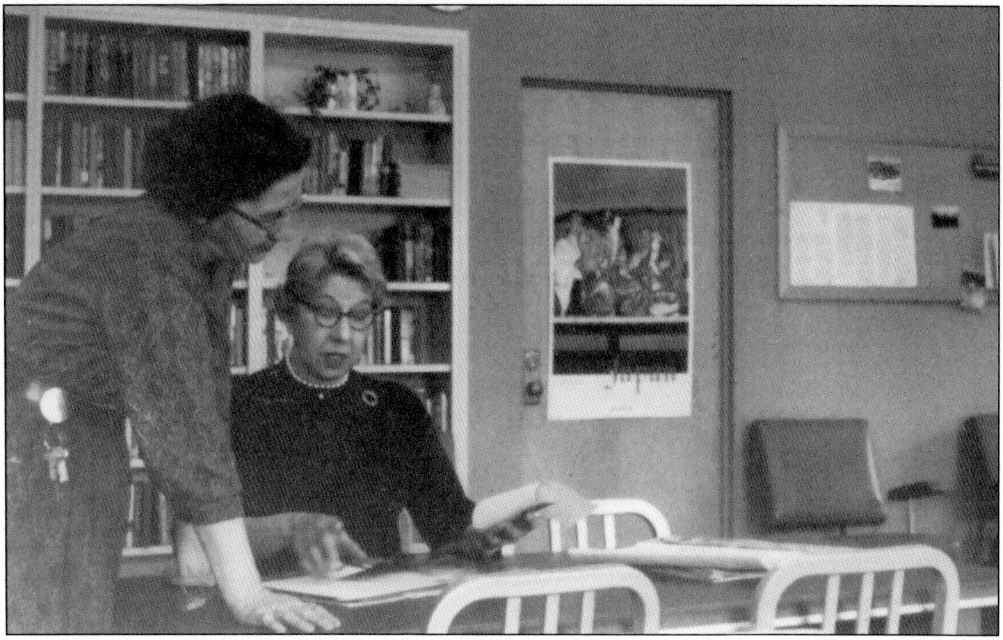

Priscilla Hill was hired in 1951 to create a library for patients. Over the years, she established reading rooms in several of the patient care buildings and provided a book cart to pass through the wards. A patient, writing in 1957, praised the library for its "quiet atmosphere, away from the standard routines of hospitalization." Hill, on the left, consults with assistant librarian Christine LaSalle in the library in the Haskell Building in 1963. Hill examines what remains of the library she opened in 1952 on the fourth-floor center of the main building in the image below, taken 40 years later, shortly before the hospital closed. Stan Sherer, a documentary photographer, took a number of photographs of employees and retired employees in their old work settings in that year. (Below, courtesy of Stan Sherer.)

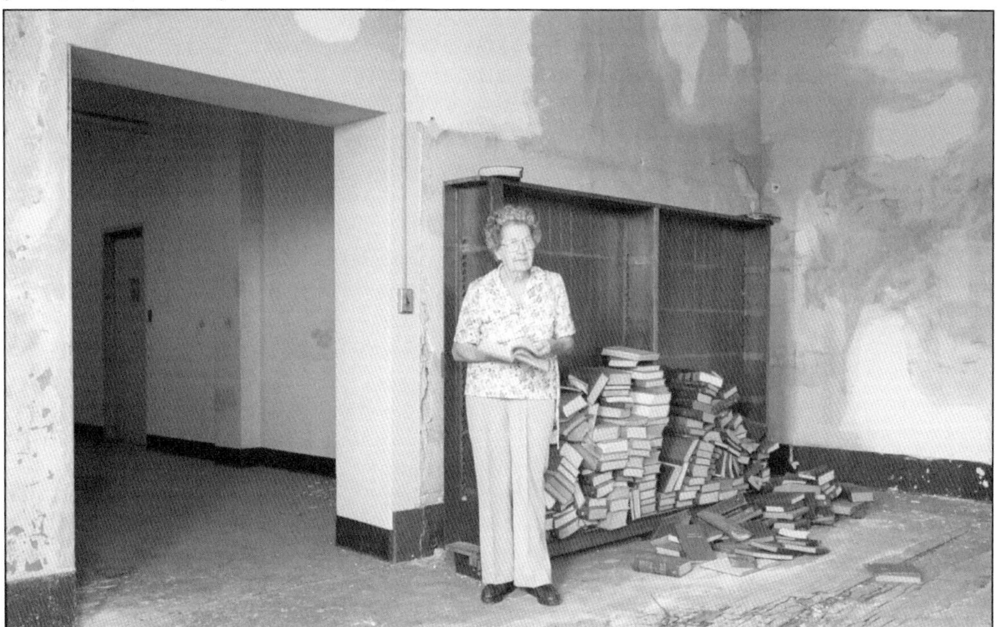

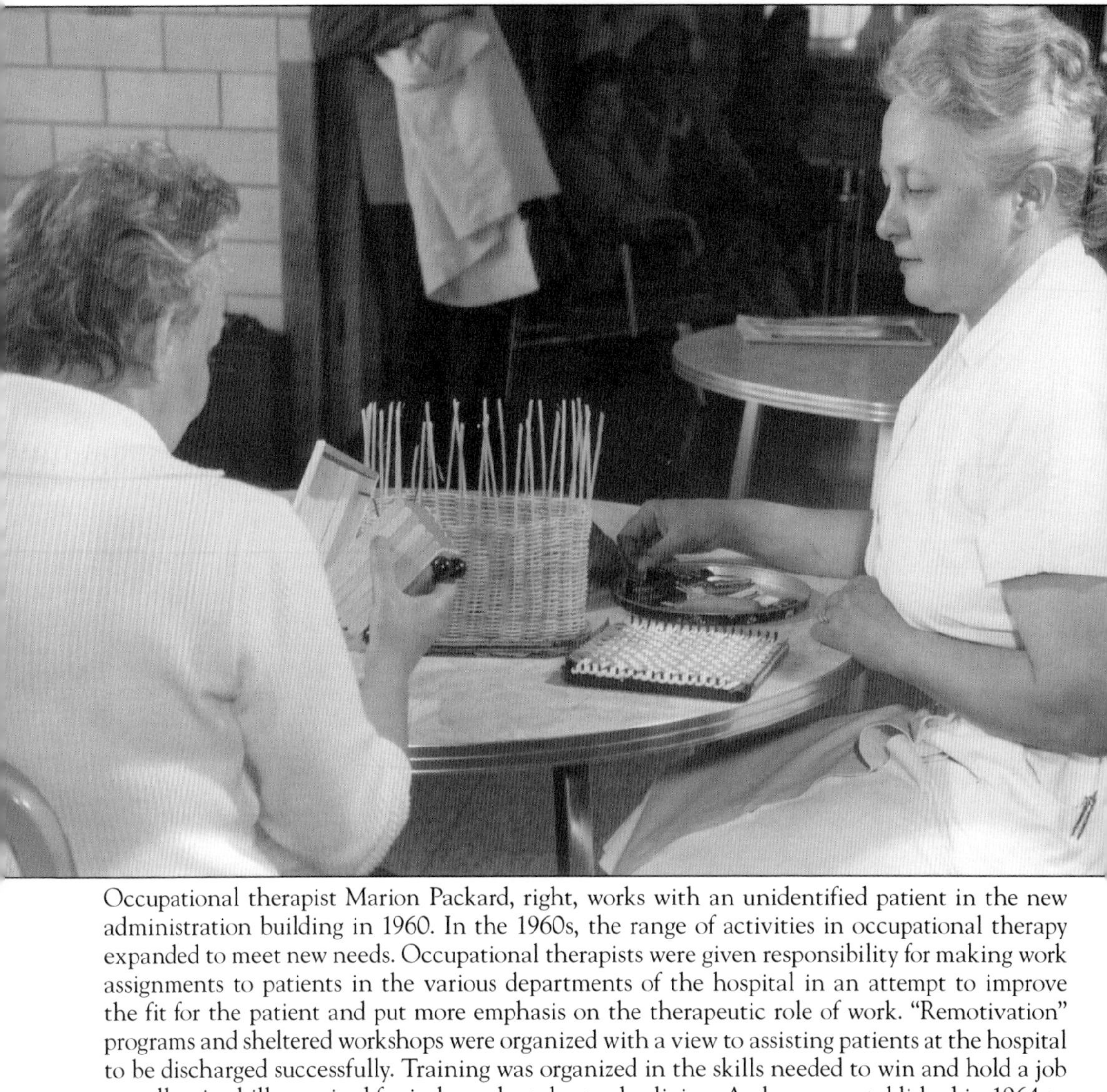

Occupational therapist Marion Packard, right, works with an unidentified patient in the new administration building in 1960. In the 1960s, the range of activities in occupational therapy expanded to meet new needs. Occupational therapists were given responsibility for making work assignments to patients in the various departments of the hospital in an attempt to improve the fit for the patient and put more emphasis on the therapeutic role of work. "Remotivation" programs and sheltered workshops were organized with a view to assisting patients at the hospital to be discharged successfully. Training was organized in the skills needed to win and hold a job as well as in skills required for independent day-to-day living. A class was established in 1964 to teach patients to become nurse's aides. A music therapy program was created. The 1970s saw the creation of movement, dance, and art therapies.

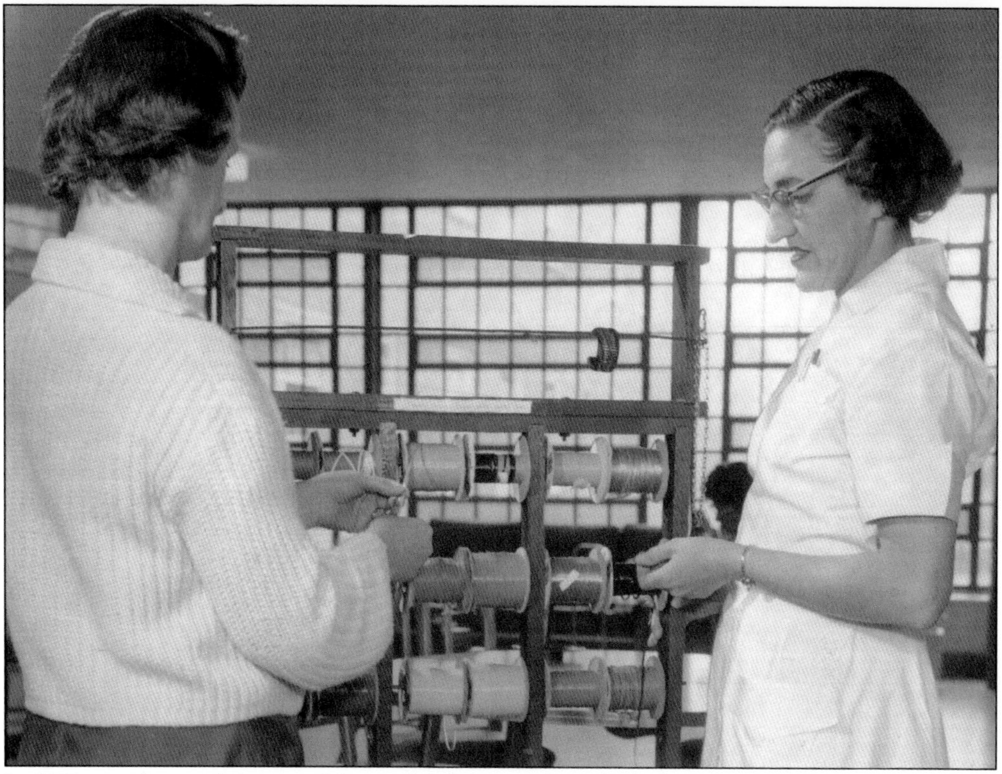

In 1960, occupational therapist Virginia Murphy, on the right, helps an unidentified patient choose materials for making a plastic place mat in the new administration building (to be renamed Haskell Building). Murphy joined the staff in 1949, after teaching school for six years. She found the work "so much more rewarding" than teaching. Intending to stay only a short time, she stayed on long term and retired after 33 years. Below, Murphy visited the room where she had led group cooking classes for patients as part of the occupational therapy department in 1992. When she started in the late 1940s, occupational therapy provided activities like crocheting and knitting for patients who could not do more active work in the departments of the hospital. As the hospital changed to offer more active treatments, her job entailed leading group therapy sessions and teaching life skills to patients before their discharge. (Below, courtesy of Stan Sherer.)

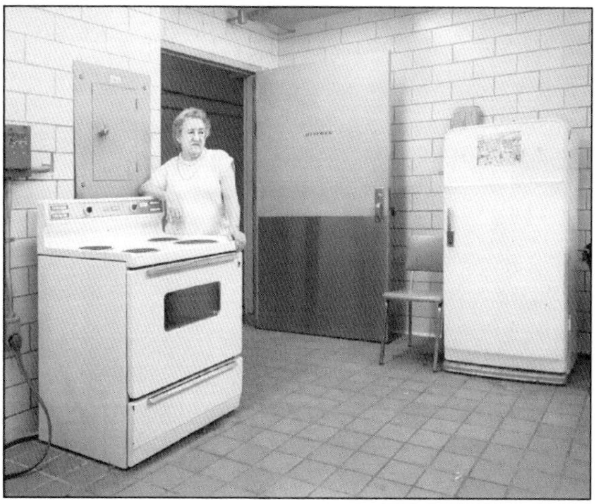

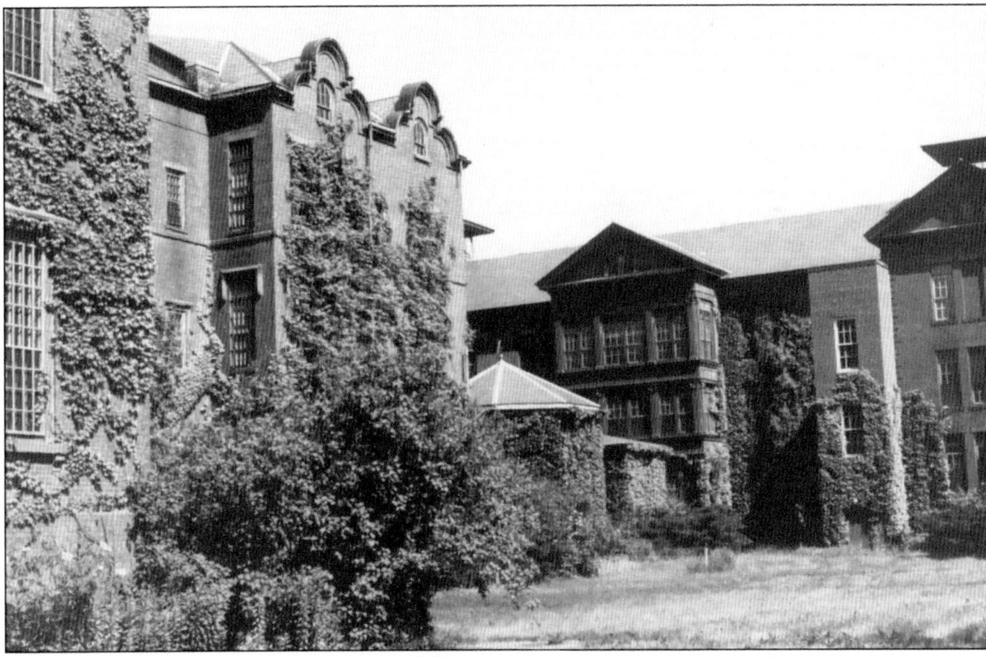

Superintendent Goodman pleaded the following in 1965: "We have buildings that have served for over 100 years, and we cannot expect them to be useful for another 100 years. Our citizens should receive better facilities than we are now offering them. These buildings are obsolete and a fire hazard, and for many years we have pointed out the danger and requested their replacement. We again beseech the authorities to heed our request for the protection of the persons entrusted in our care."

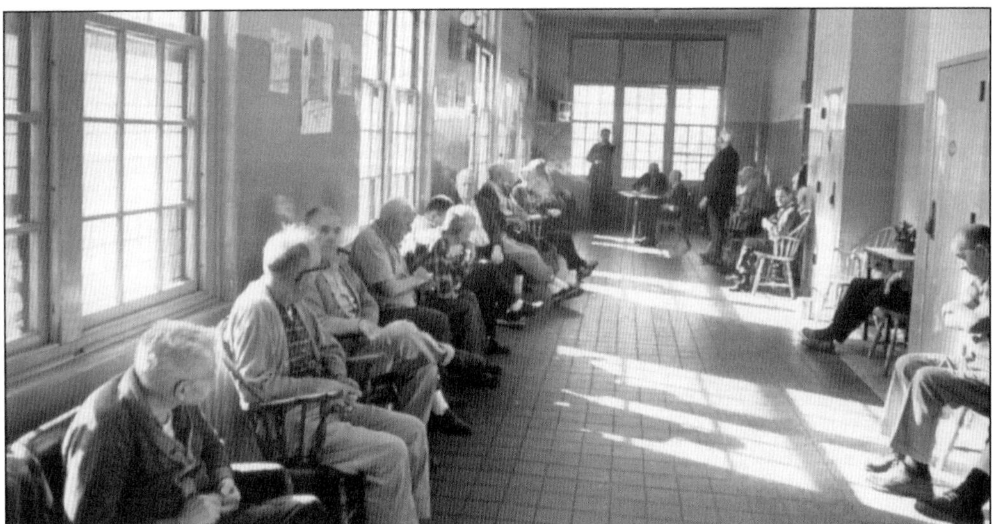

"Public Indifference Blamed for Present Deplorable Conditions in Massachusetts Mental Institutions." This photograph of the dayroom ran with that headline in a newspaper in 1967. A year earlier, a community-based system of mental health care was mandated by federal law. Even so, the state hospitals remained the main site of care for clients for years to come. Over the next two decades, the situation worsened, as the state grew more reluctant to put money into hospitals they intended to close. This is the same dayroom shown in the photograph on page 51.

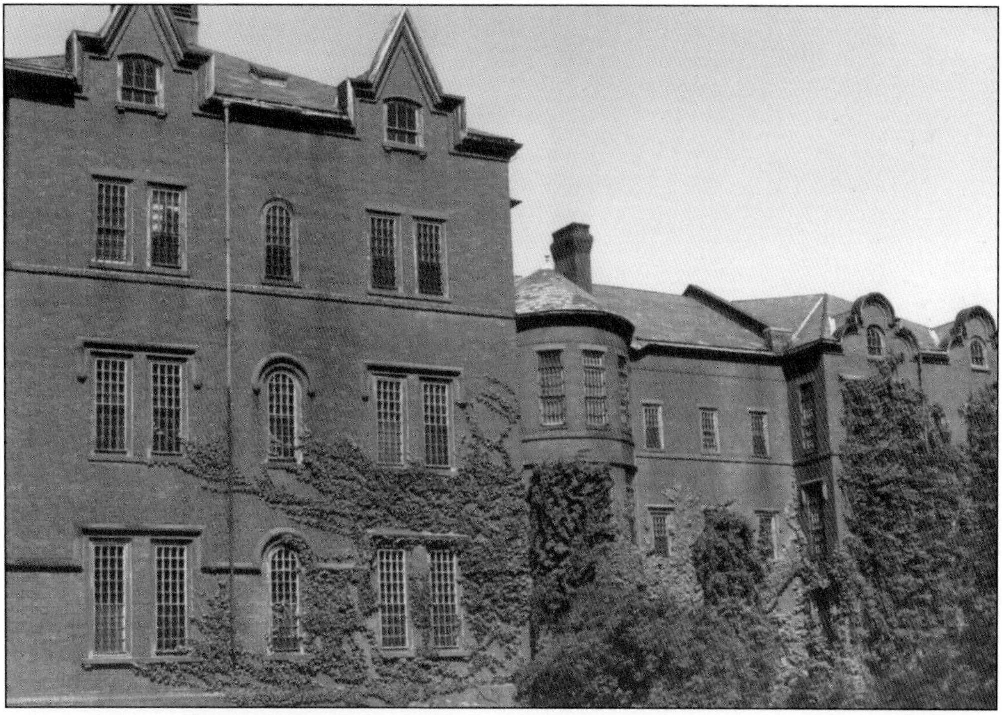

"The state hospital very seldom turned anyone away from its doors. It has that charm about it, it seems to want to draw you in, like a bear hug. I met my fair share of Christs and Political Prisoners while I was at Northampton State Hospital," remembers a former patient. "The boredom was emotionally draining. I remember the night a girl in tears told me that she was certain her brain was dying."

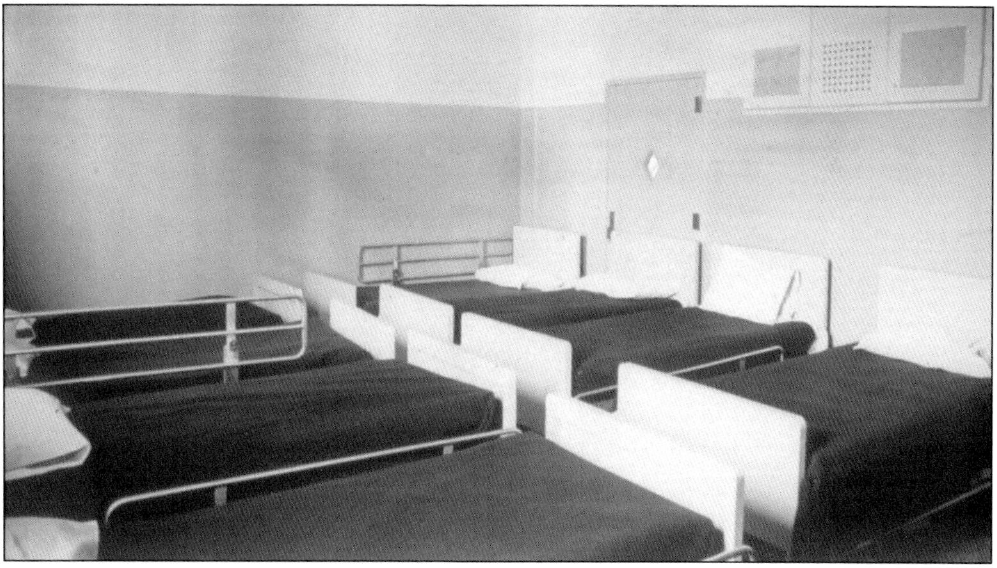

Shown here is an impossibly cramped dormitory in the main building in 1967. Not only is there virtually no room to get in and out of bed, but also one of the exits is clearly blocked. The hospital publicized its many needs at this time in hopes of galvanizing public support for greater funding.

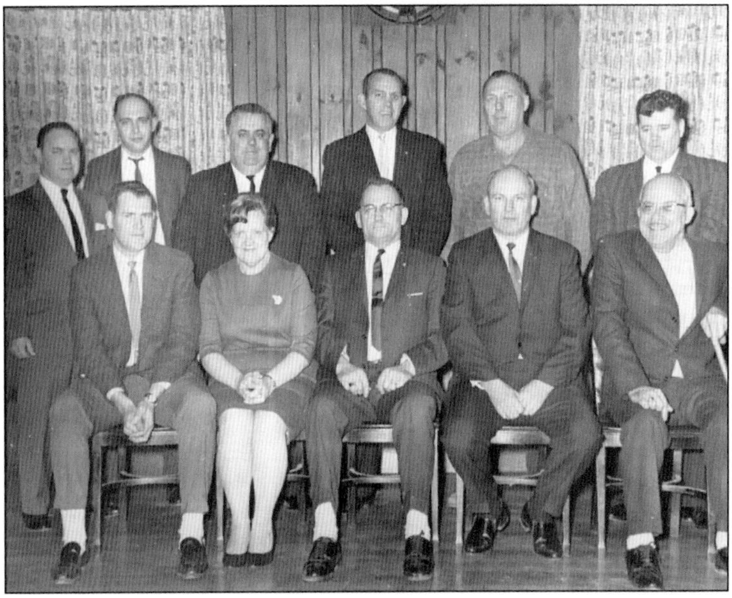

Massachusetts state workers won the right to collectively bargain in 1964. The licensed practical nurses, service personnel, and later, the ward attendants organized in the American Federation of State, County, and Municipal Employees (AFSCME) Local No. 165. Local leaders gathered here with union officials.

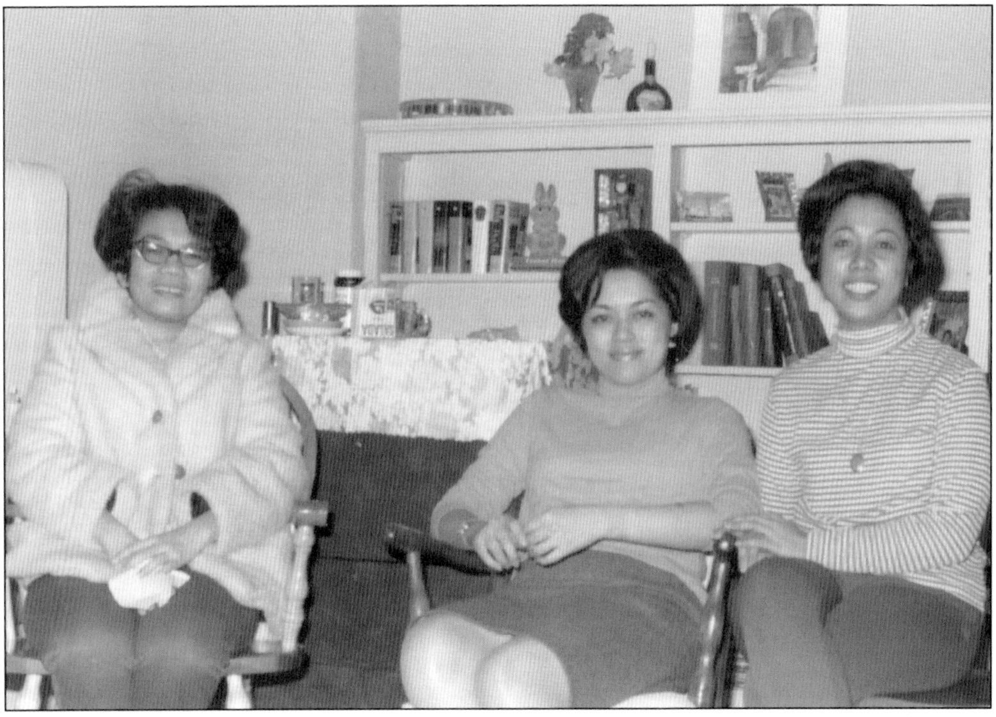

Drs. Rina Belen, Malu Benemerito, and Leonor Pagtakan are seen from left to right in this 1969 snapshot. At this time, foreign-trained doctors were allowed to practice at the hospital using temporary licenses under the supervision of a board-certified doctor. Often, these doctors were not trained in psychiatry. When the state stopped honoring temporary licenses in 1977, the hospital contracted with other institutions for medical services, starting with the University of Massachusetts Medical School.

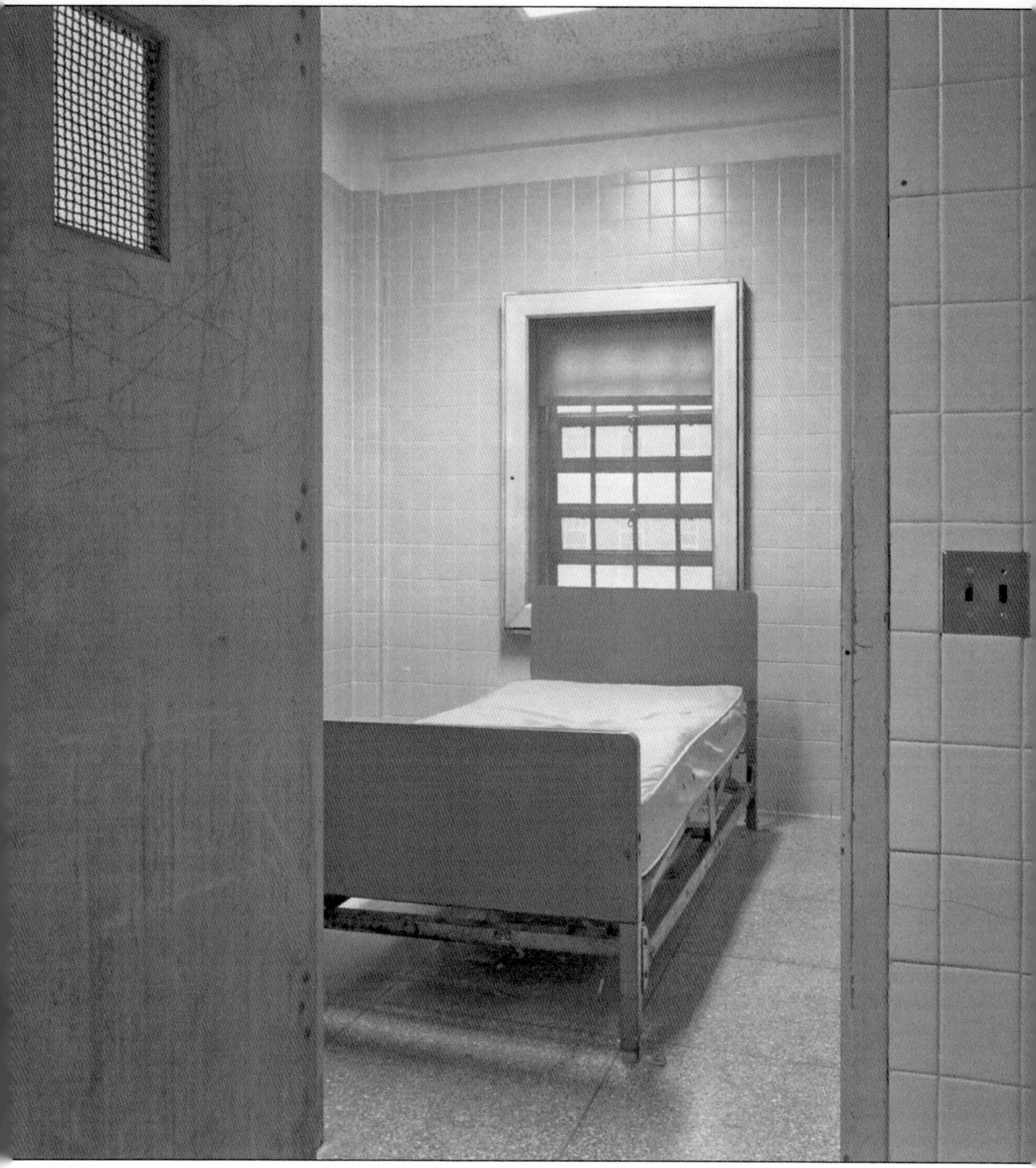

"How one is supposed to conduct themselves on a state hospital ward, that all depends on how bad you want to get out. I never met very many patients who liked seclusion, much less how they were brought in. Many would do whatever they could do to fight, including kick, punch, or bite. You have to understand how patients thought about being pushed around. It wasn't in our nature to go peacefully. I think it's human nature," reported a former patient. Here is a seclusion room in the G Building, opened in 1969 as a medical building. It was converted to a center of general patient care as the census declined and the main buildings were vacated by 1975. The tile walls, metal fixtures, and large wards offering little privacy made it a less-than-ideal location for mental health treatment. (Courtesy of Stan Sherer.)

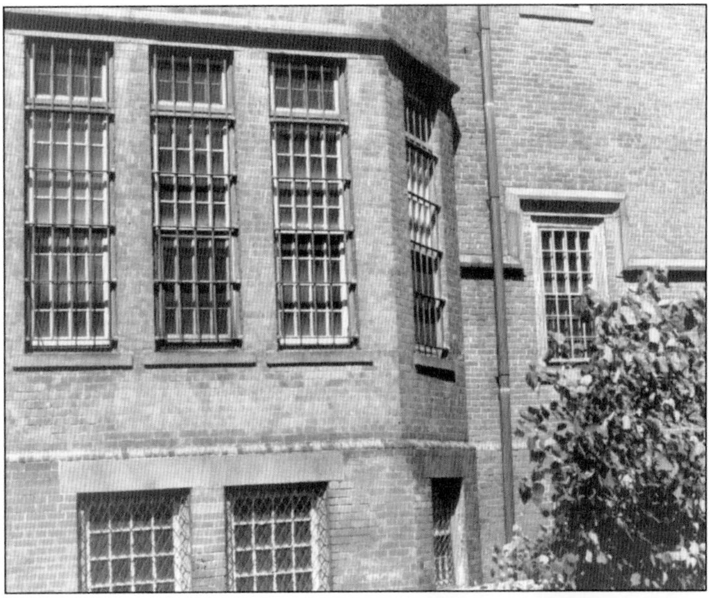

In 1957, patient R. La Chance's poem "Heart on the Hill" was published in the hospital's then new literary journal: "Outside Doors / A little fresh air / And a whole lot more / Just outside that locked door. / Not for you, not for me. / We are locked in you see. / Oh! just to get that key. / For outside that door is a little fresh air / And a whole lot more."

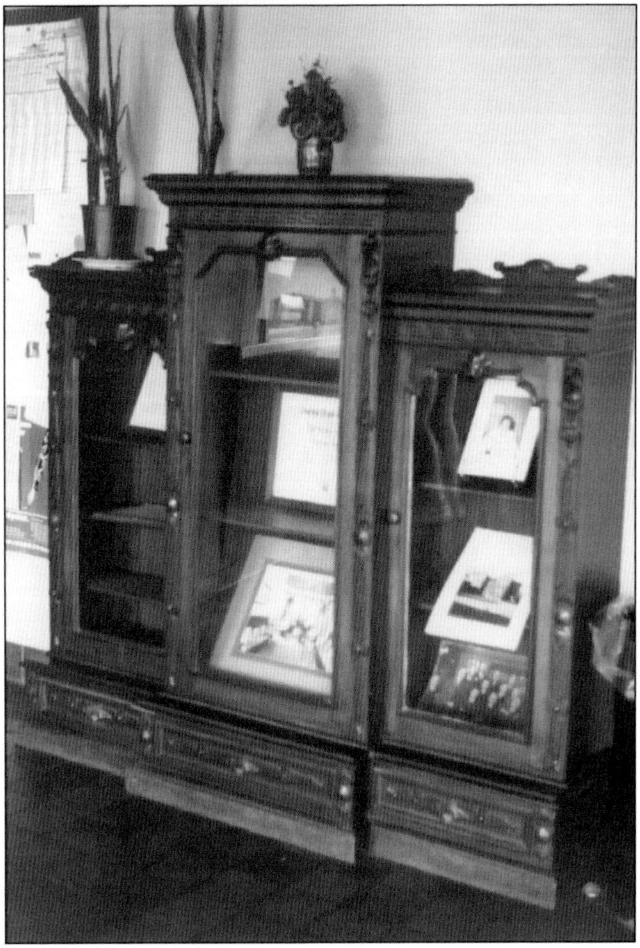

The hospital tried to keep track of its own history in bits and pieces, with most of the original furniture and records changing locations multiple times—from the old main building to Haskell Building and then on to other places. The Massachusetts State Archives in Boston has been the main receptacle of documents from closing state hospitals; more than 40,000 unsorted boxes of records and documents are stored off-site in a warehouse, waiting to be accessed.

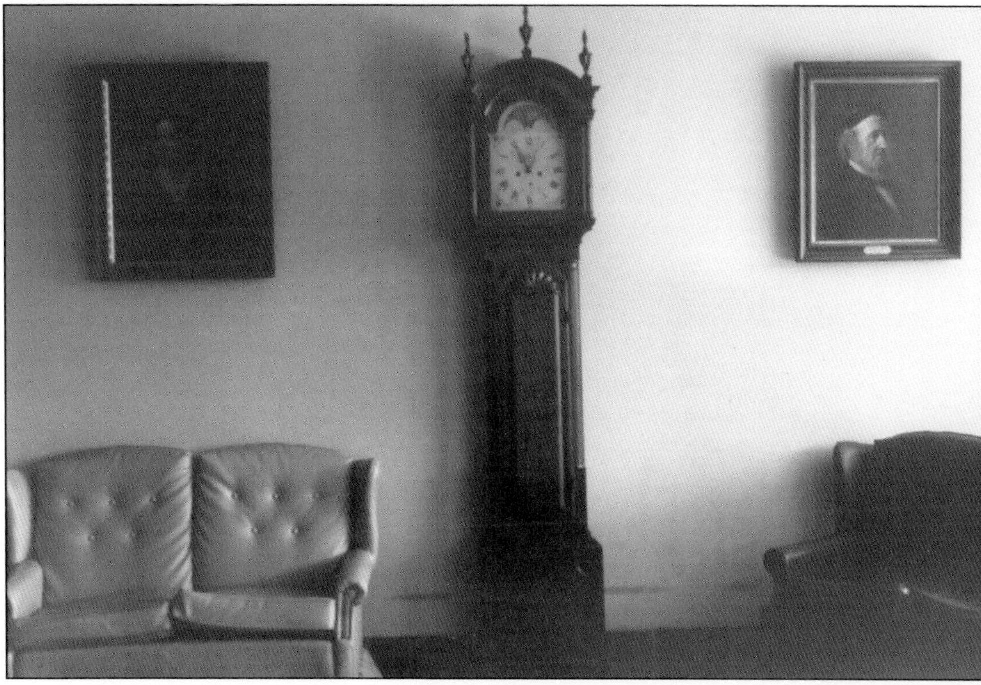

Pictured above is a room on the first floor of the Haskell Building. As the wooden furniture from the 19th century dwindled and got replaced by metal chairs and beds, some of the original treasures survive to this day, like the painted portraits of Dorothea Dix and of Pliny Earle flanking the exquisite clock that was an Earle family heirloom. Pliny Earle presented the clock as a gift to the hospital on May 5, 1887, while he lived there in retirement. It dates back to 1800 and was made by David Williams in Newport, Rhode Island.

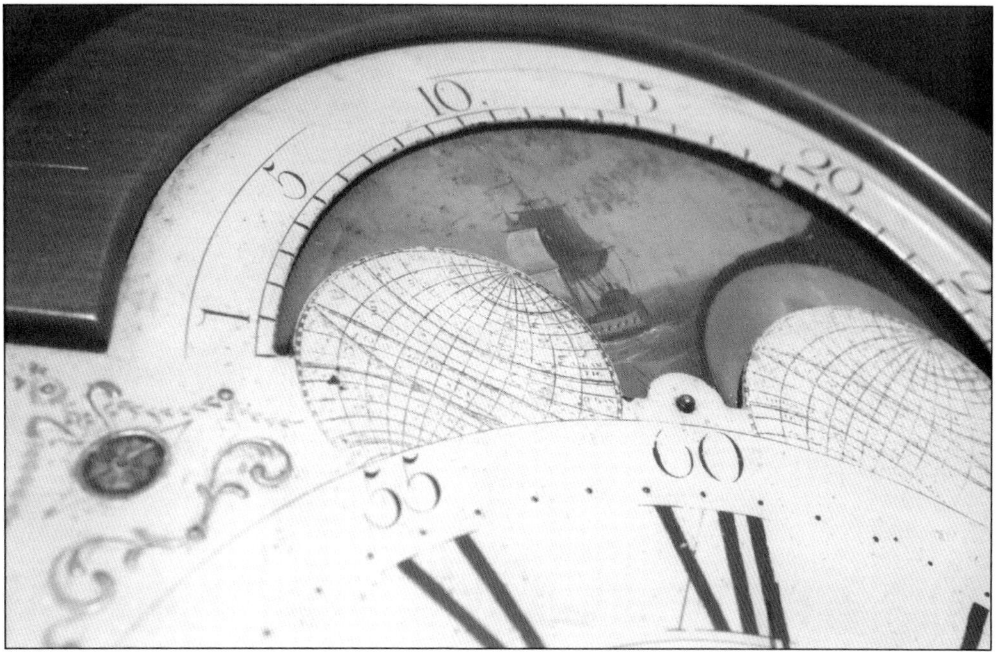

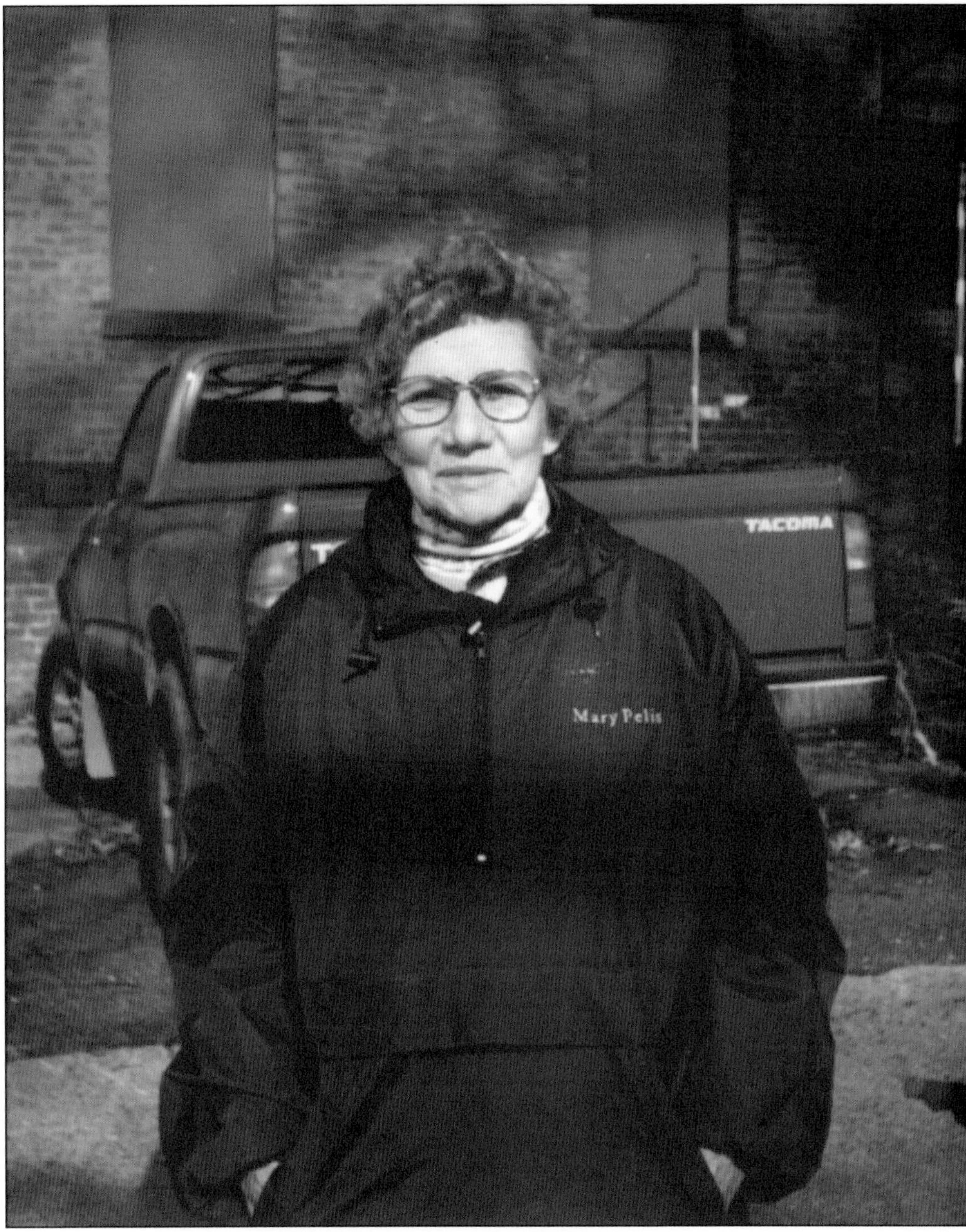

The vast numbers of elderly patients were a great challenge at state hospitals. Between 1970 and 1975, the "geriatric care team" placed more than 800 patients into the community. Created by Eaton and staffed by six highly committed and skilled nurses and social workers, whole new strategies had to be invented for placements of patients into the community. "You place them only where I'd place my own mother, I always told those nurses. That's all," remembers Eaton. But it was not an easy task. "We were doing things that had no template, we didn't have something to compare it against, except itself," said Department of Mental Health area director James Duffy. Longtime employee Mary Pelis, RN, shown here in her volunteer windbreaker during "Habeas Corpus," a sound installation, in 2000, personally placed more than 400 people into nursing homes, rest homes, and other community settings. (Courtesy of Katherine Turman.)

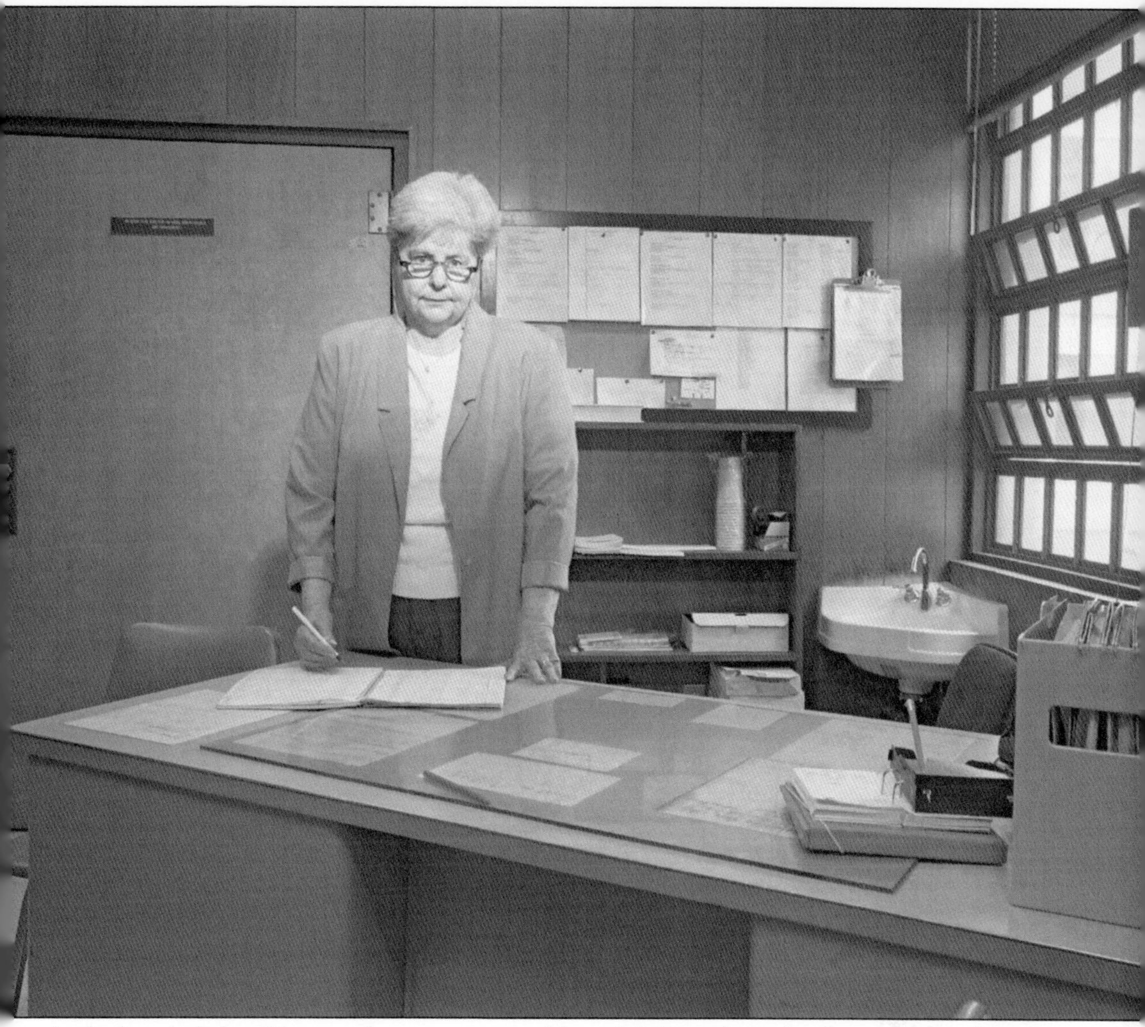

In the hospital's last 20 years, there were many able and dedicated people who worked to change the hospital and develop an effective system of community care and treatment. In the 1970s, many nurses and social workers trained for work in the community. People like Betty Reed, RN, straddled the two worlds of the hospital and the community. She transferred from the hospital to the Westfield area, creating programs and housing for former patients. Several years later, she returned to the hospital as an area director. The Reed House, a group home in Westfield, is named in her honor. She is shown here in the old offices of the geriatric care team. (Courtesy of Stan Sherer.)

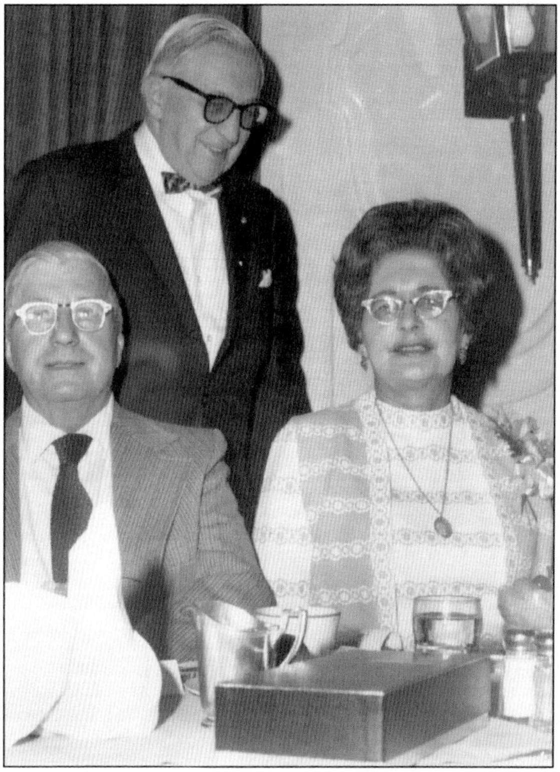

When Dr. Harry Goodman took over the reins of leadership in 1958, the hospital looked and operated much as it had for the previous 50 years. When he retired in 1973, the hospital was fundamentally changed. During his time as superintendent, the hospital was reorganized to provide more active patient treatment, and hundreds were successfully relocated into community residences. Here, Goodman and his wife receive congratulations at his retirement party from assistant commissioner Wilfred Bloomberg.

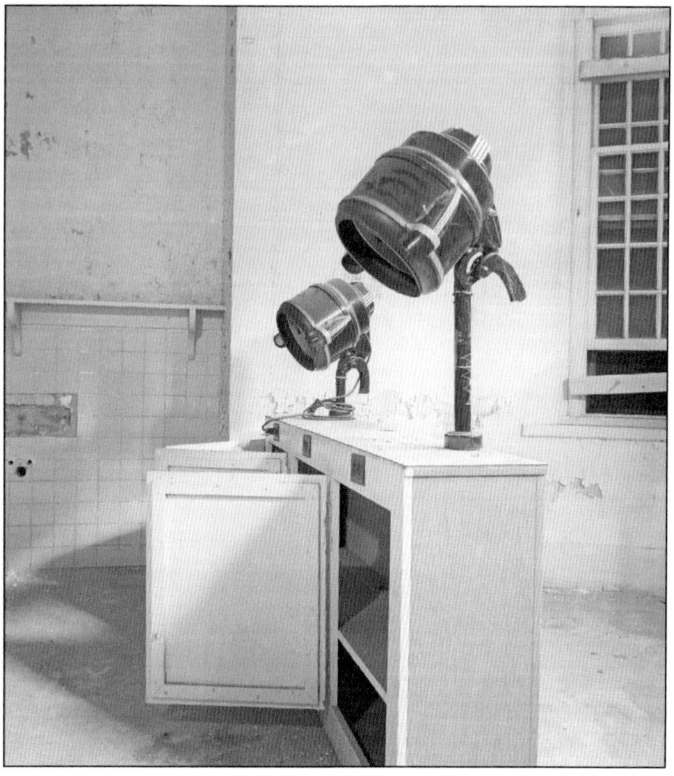

"The opening of a beauty parlor on the female service on October 27, 1952, has had remarkable results in the rehabilitation of women patients," reads an annual report. Betty Heald, the last hospital hairdresser, said, "They enjoyed it because they were getting personal attention. I would listen to their stories and talk to them. I wasn't judging them; I was giving them the treatment." (Courtesy of Stan Sherer.)

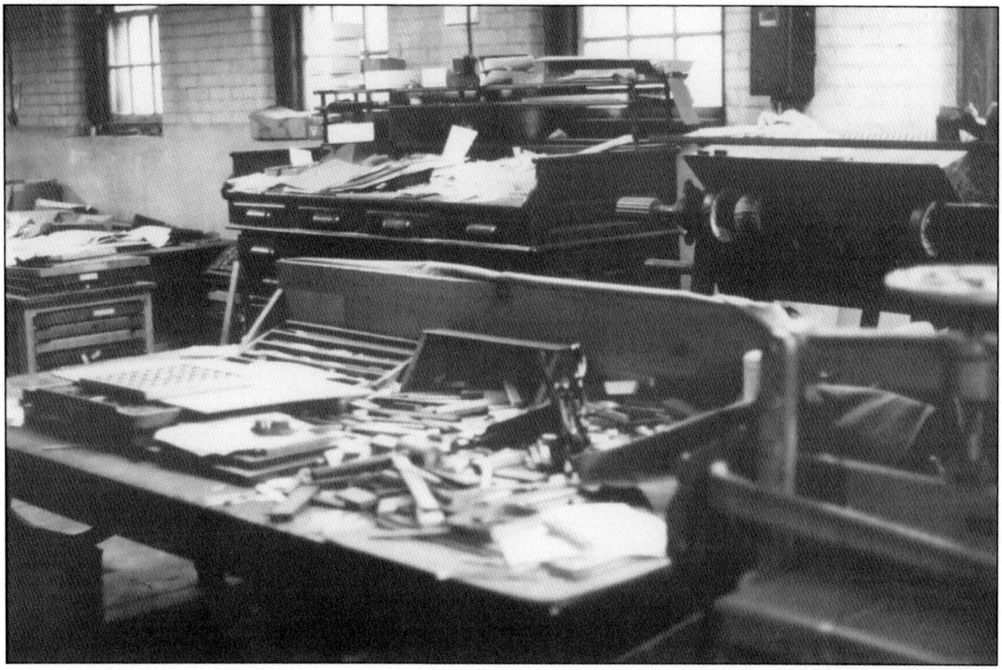

The bookbindery in the basement of C Building, shown above, was where all of the reports for the state hospitals were bound for many years. When Bob Elliott was in charge in the 1960s and 1970s, he sometimes had as many as a dozen patients working there at one time. The shoe shop, below, was also a very productive place, patching, soling, or heeling hundreds of pairs of shoes each year. These images, however, convey obsolescence and decay. As historical activities of the hospital were discontinued, room after room was abandoned, and it appeared as if everyone had just locked the door and walked away.

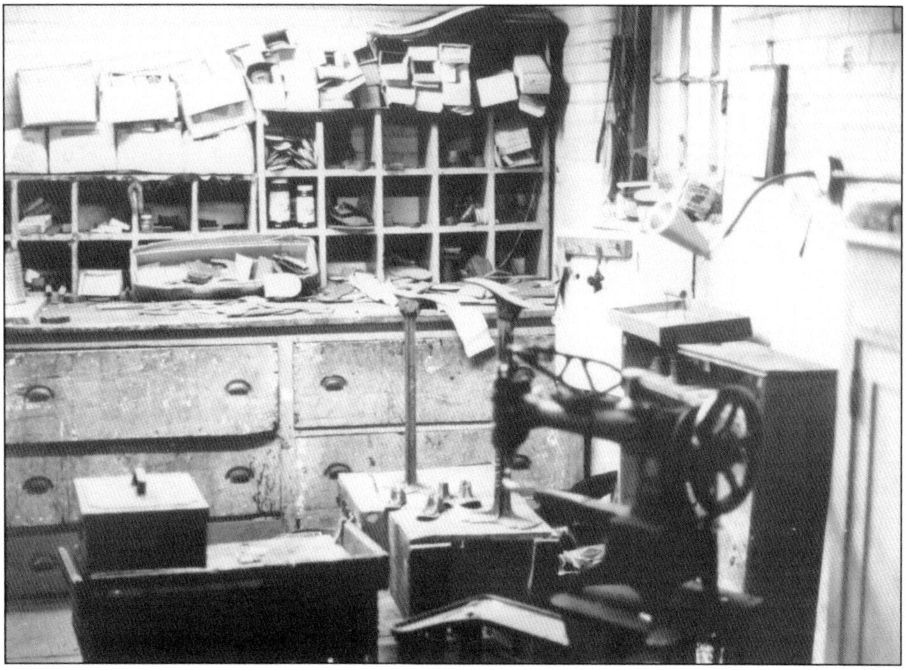

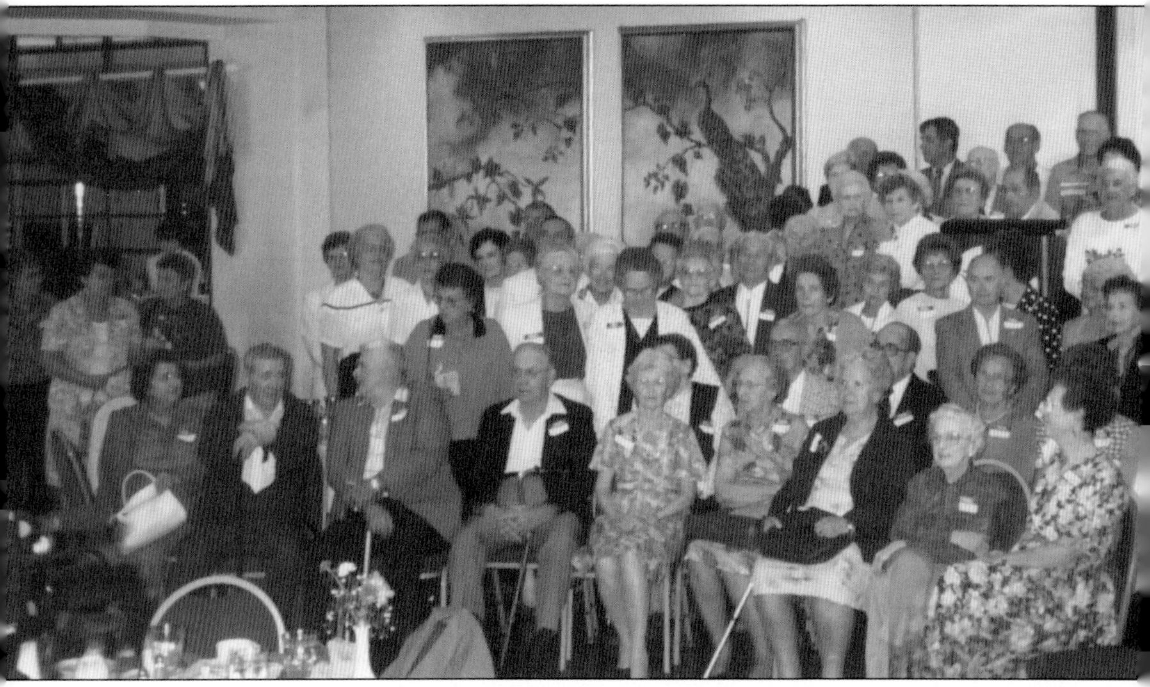

More than 200 retired hospital workers and their friends gathered for a reunion in 1992, a few months before the hospital closed after 135 years in service. Their memories of "hospital hill" reached back all the way to 1920. They had worked in every capacity, from gardener and ward attendant to nursing director and superintendent. Some lived their whole lives in the

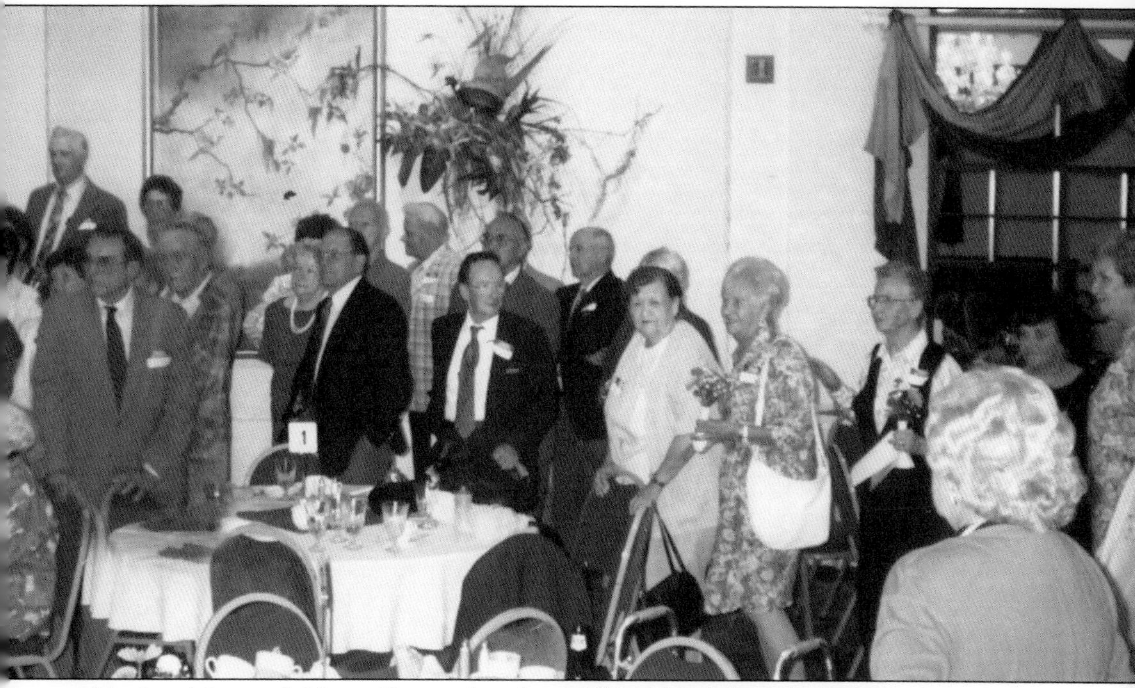

neighborhood, being children of hospital workers. All had lived through the large changes that reshaped the mental health care system and brought the hospital from a facility housing 2,500 patients to one on the verge of permanent closure.

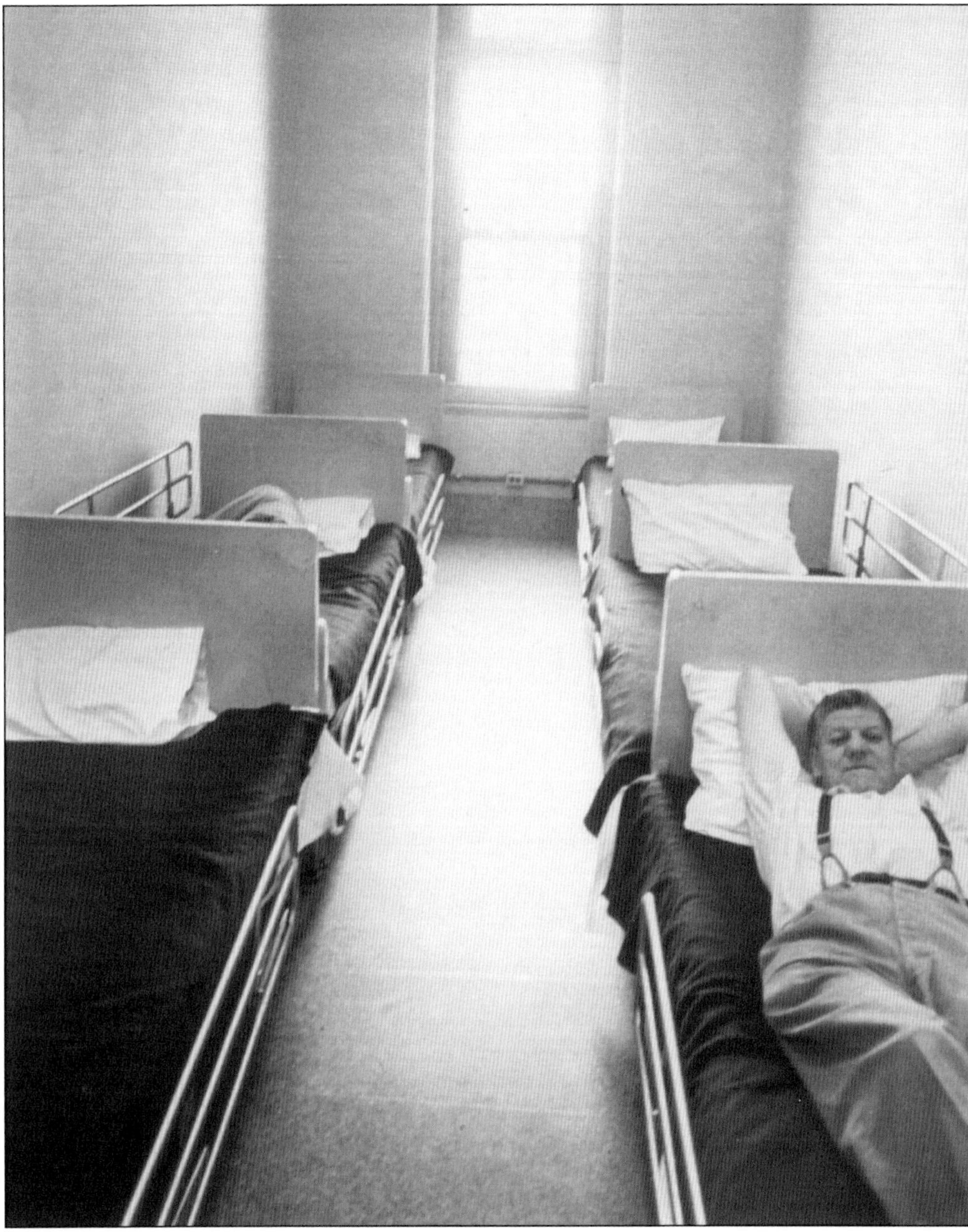

After three years of working with patients in the hospital to enforce their legal and civil rights, the Mental Patients Advocacy Project (MPAP) won a lawsuit in 1975 establishing that before a court in Massachusetts can commit a person with mental illness, it must consider whether there is a less restrictive alternative to involuntary hospitalization. A year later, MPAP filed a landmark class-action lawsuit, *Brewster v. Dukakis*, on their behalf. It claimed that the state's failure to provide them with community-based alternatives to the hospital violated their constitutional rights. A consent decree was entered into in 1978, guaranteeing the establishment of a comprehensive community mental health system in the area served by the hospital. A federal judge would oversee this process, which took much longer than expected and hit many snags along the way. The people in this late-1960s photograph are unidentified.

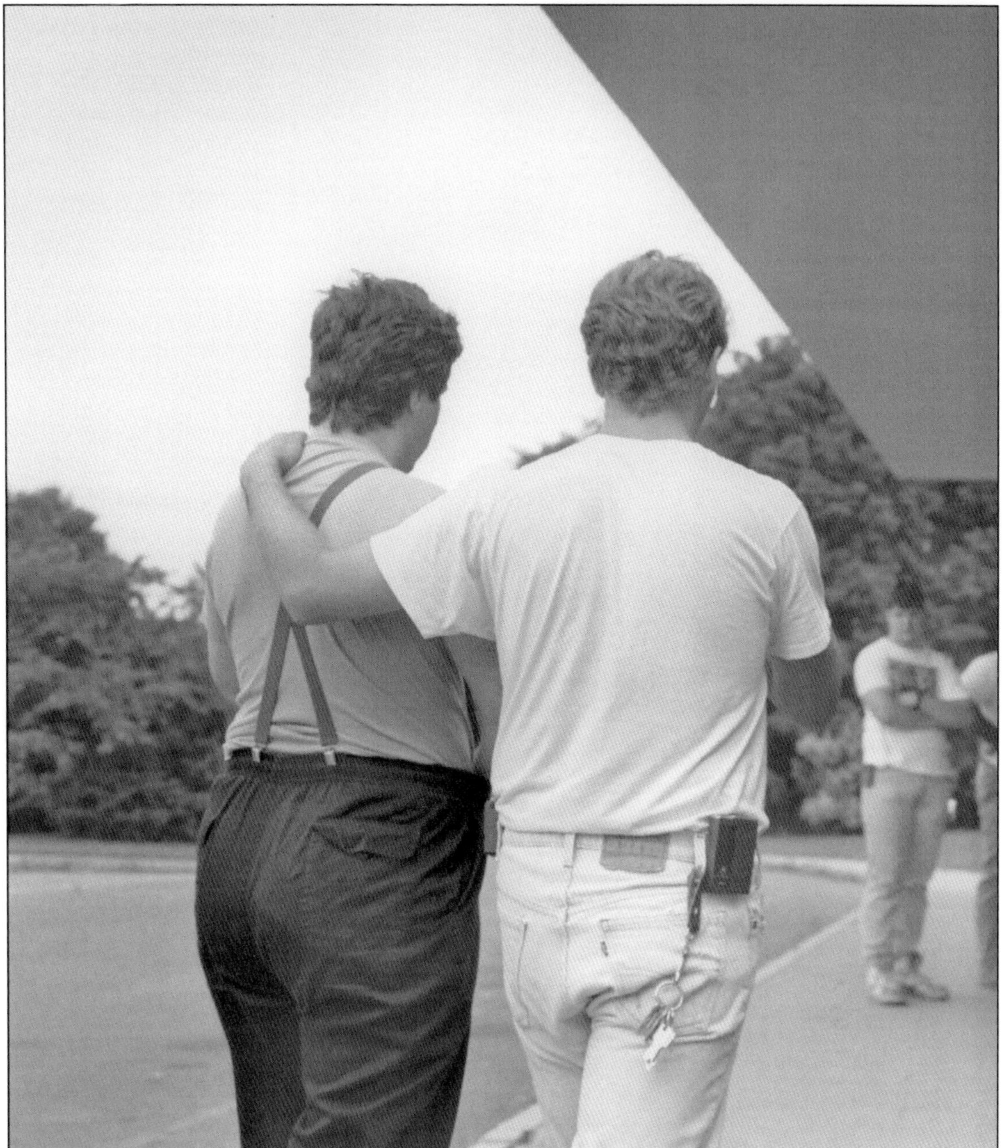

The consent decree forced the state to create a system of community-based care. As this system developed, the census at the hospital declined. Nearly 700 new "beds" were created in the community by 1986, and every person in the hospital when the consent decree was signed was eventually placed out. More than half avoided readmission to the hospital, though for younger people with histories of frequent hospitalizations, staying out of the hospital was more difficult. The optimism of the movement for community treatment was tempered by this challenge, and the need for a hospital was apparent. Even so, the state closed the hospital in a cost-cutting measure, and the capacity of municipal hospitals was expanded to meet the need. Now, mental health services are dispersed across the region, with facilities from North Adams to Greenfield to Springfield. In a major change in direction, the state also now funds several consumer-run programs, such as the Recovery Learning Center in Holyoke. Here, a staff member escorts a patient into the Haskell Building as part of the last of many consolidations of the wards at the hospital in 1993. (Courtesy of Stan Sherer.)

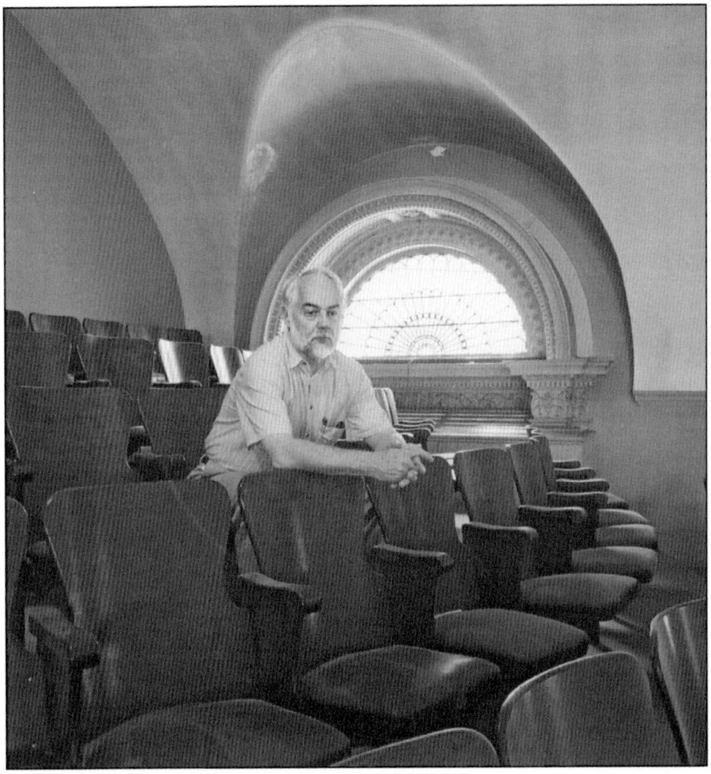

George Button Jr. organized and ran a music therapy program in the 1960s, making recorded and live music available to patients and directing theatrical productions. Later, he became an occupational therapist, retiring as the director of rehabilitation when the hospital closed. As the hospital was slated for closure, he led a committee of employees that documented its history. His father, George Sr., is shown on page 61. (Courtesy of Stan Sherer.)

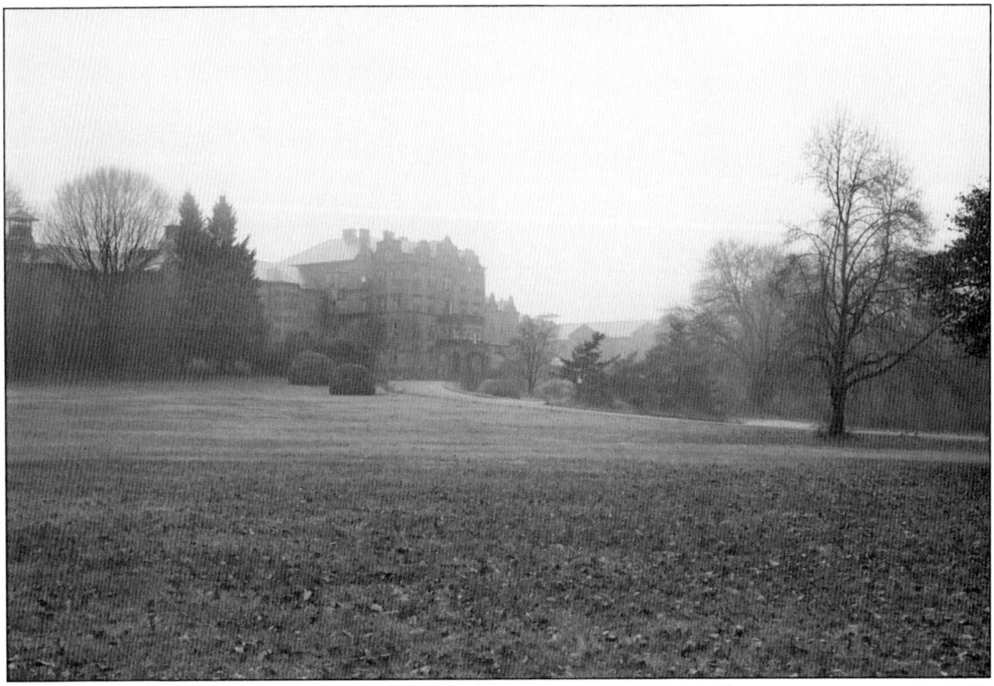

After nearly 20 years of neglect, the main buildings maintained a striking presence on the hill, fired the imagination of visitors, and prompted rumination about the lives of those who had passed through them. (Courtesy of Stan Sherer.)

Four

Remembrance

Northampton State Hospital closed more than 20 years ago. The original buildings were shuttered 40 years ago. Yet it is still alive today in the lives of countless people, and what happened there matters profoundly. People who went to work there as raw youths remember like it was yesterday incidents that happened half a century ago. A young lawyer's life course was changed by his first encounter with patients on the wards, leading to a lifetime of struggle for their rights. A mother's visit to see her son propelled her on a path that led to real power for consumers in monitoring care and treatment. Sadly, it is very difficult to discern the experience of those whose encounter with the hospital was the most profound—the more than 65,000 people who were patients here over its long history.

Northampton State Hospital was a place of suffering, despair, cruelty, and loss. And sometimes it was also a place of shelter, compassion, and hope. It is not surprising that a place of such import has been the subject of many efforts at remembrance. As the hospital prepared to close in 1993, a worker-sponsored project collected the memories of some of the people who cared deeply about the history and meaning of the hospital. A client-led effort marked the site of the graveyard where several hundred indigent and friendless patients were buried. A coalition rallied people to save the old buildings and establish a small museum in them. That effort failed, but attempts to mark the site and the things that happened there continue.

As part of a widely attended memorial effort in 2000, former patients spoke movingly to the public about their own experiences with and feelings about the place that figured so prominently in their lives. But most who were treated here over the years, behind locked doors to which they had no key, left no personal account of their experiences. Indeed, it was the nature of the hospital, during most of its history, to strip patients of their pasts when they walked through the door, leaving them unmoored and adrift. In the end, it is their silence that speaks loudest.

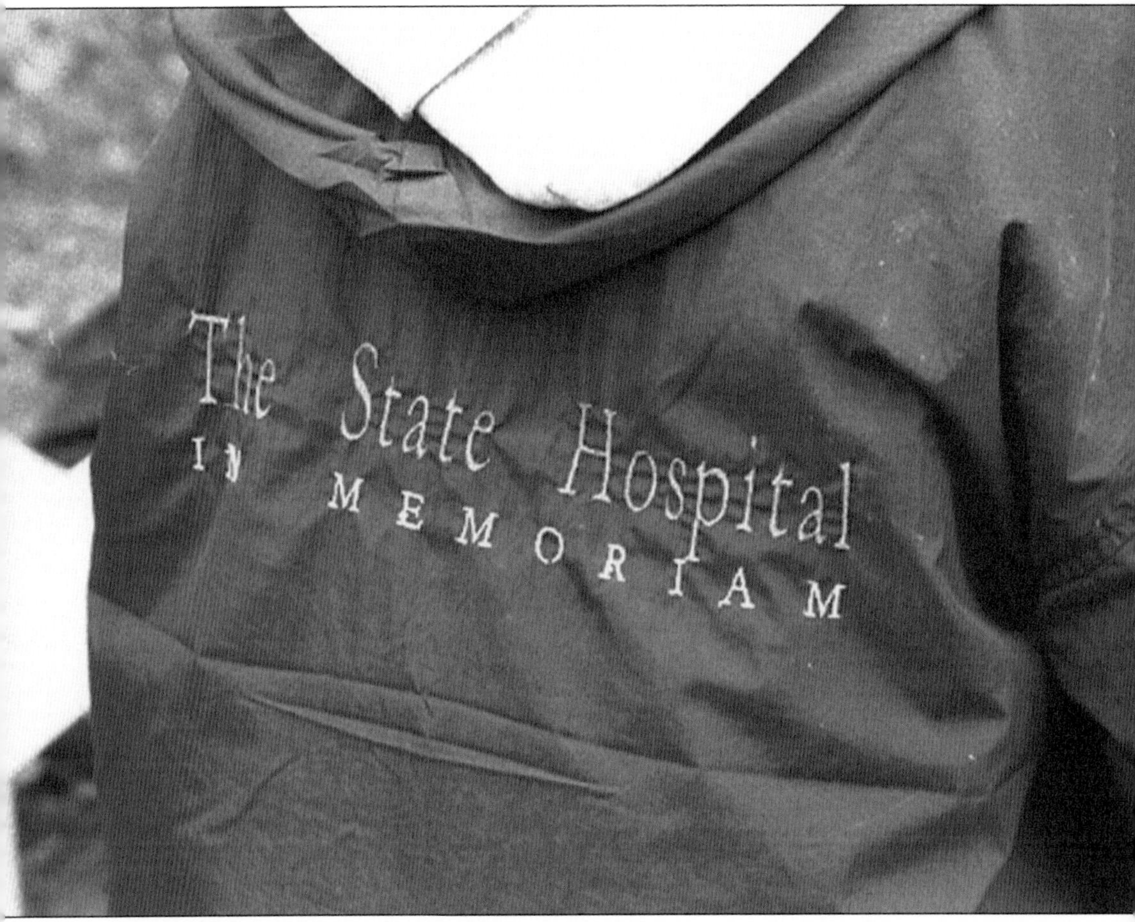

A series of memorial events took place on November 17 and 18, 2000. The events included a symposium at Smith College, with Michael Dukakis as keynote speaker, and psychiatrists from around the United States as panelists, followed by three exhibitions in town, including one at the Anchor House of Artists, a studio and arts-support group run by and for artists diagnosed with serious mental illness. An open forum took place the following morning, during which former patients shared their stories of the hospital openly and freely to a packed audience. The forum was followed by the ringing of church bells and a citywide moment of silence, as thousands walked up to the hospital and gathered around the old main building for "Habeas Corpus," a sound installation. (Courtesy of Hedwig Schüßler.)

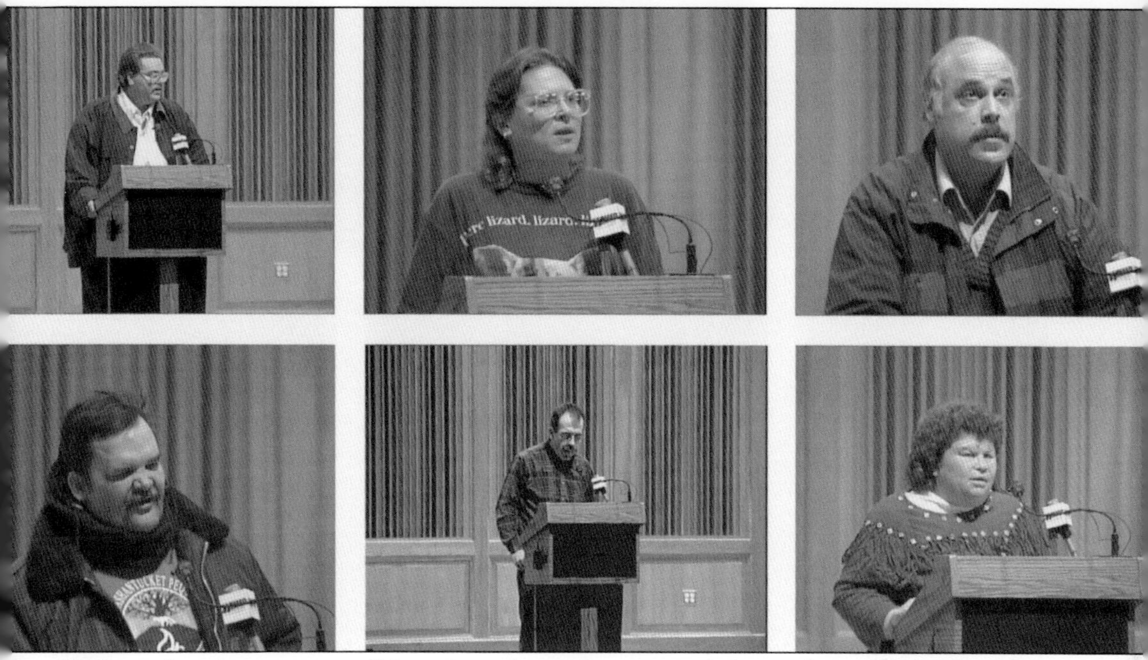

"With profound respect we will hear from those who intimately know about the Northampton State Hospital—from the inside" were the words with which Steven Schwartz welcomed the audience to the open forum. As an attorney, he founded the Center for Public Representation in the 1970s to provide legal assistance to patients at Northampton State Hospital. He filed a class-action lawsuit on their behalf and continued to work with them until the hospital closed. The forum offered an opportunity for former patients, several of whom are pictured above, to speak the truth about their experiences at Northampton State Hospital. David Petersen made a short film about this day. (Courtesy of Hedwig Schüßler.)

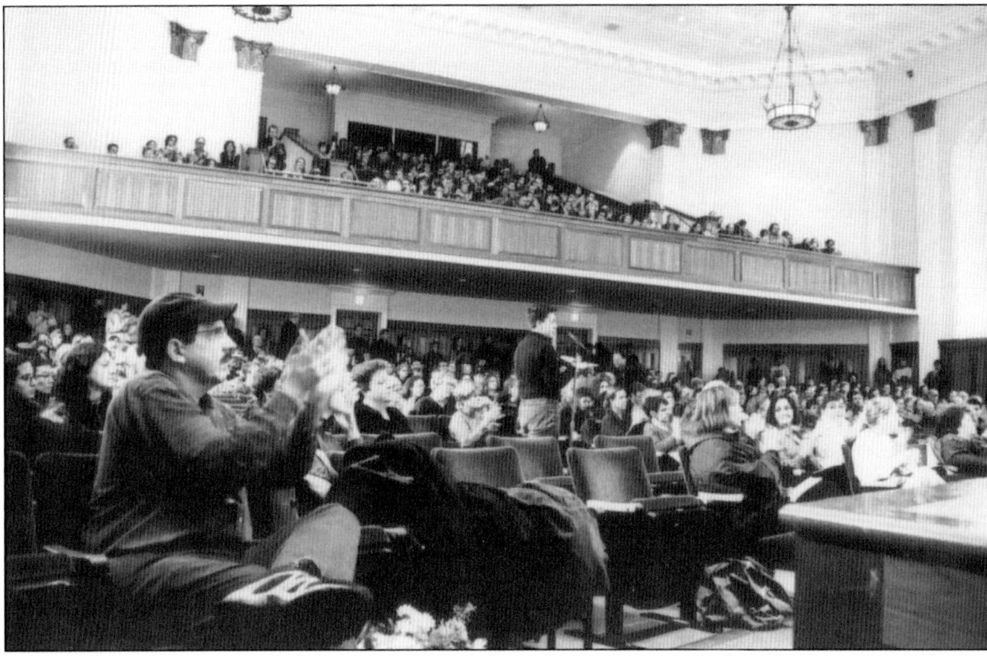

In addition to the testimonies, a "Pledge of Remembrance and Welcoming" was read at the forum, which the audience was invited to share, and it stated, "For the thousands of mental patients who have resided in state hospitals, for those long dead, for those still living and surviving: Promise to Remember." It ended with "we promise to remember to welcome people labeled mentally ill into our affirming communities and to join together to build a better today and an even more promising tomorrow for everyone. And so may it be." On the morning of the memorial events, an aerial photograph was taken, showing the immense main building as it was wired up with sound. Over the course of its history, the building had grown to over 414,000 square feet of continuous indoor space. (Above, courtesy of Hedwig Schüßler; below, courtesy of Paul Franz.)

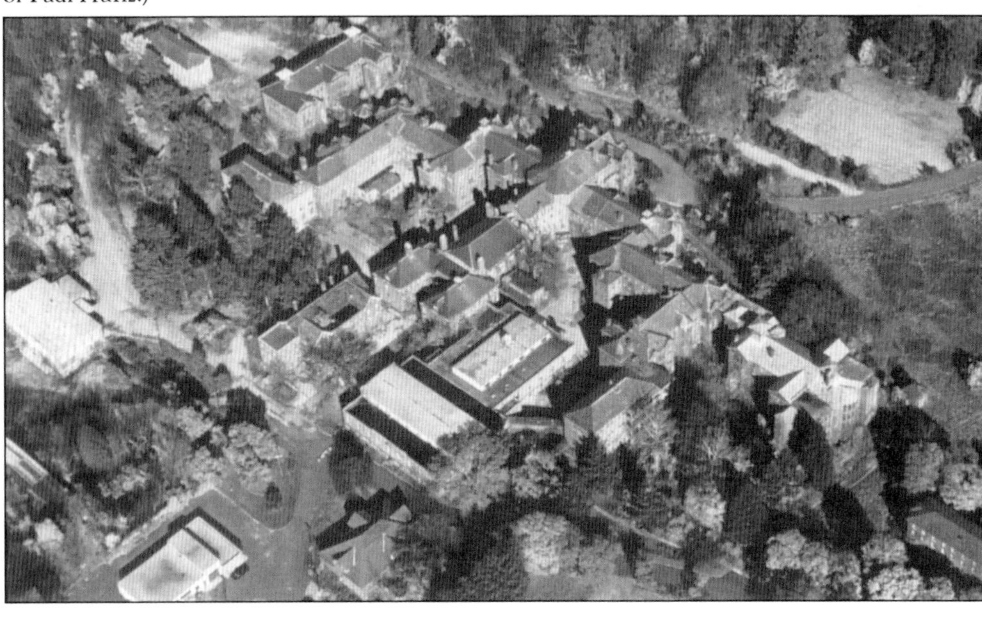

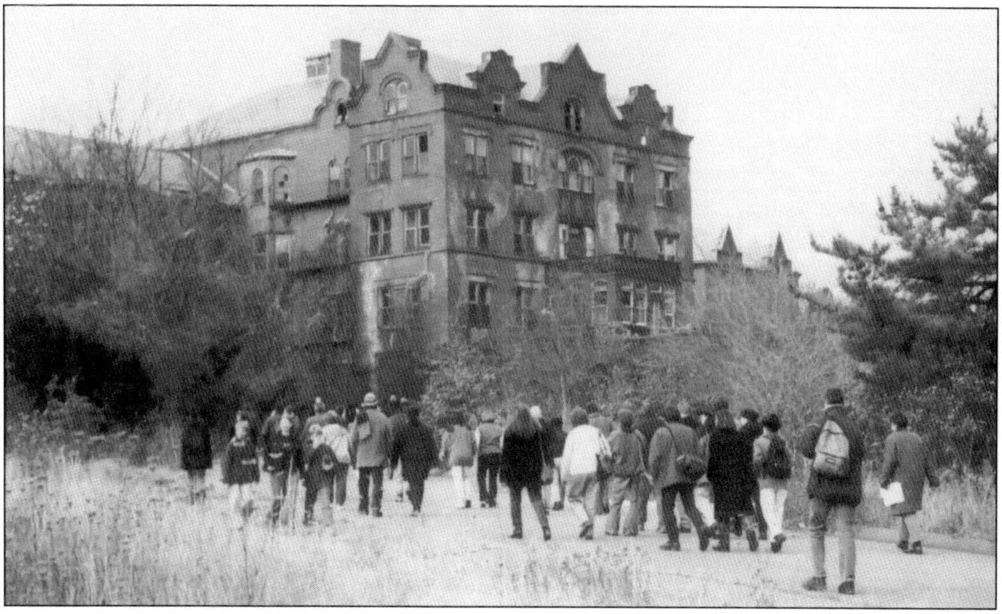

Following the open forum—and in reference to the laying of the cornerstone in 1856, when the public made a lengthy parade up the hospital hill—the public was invited to walk up the hill once more to gather at the hospital and to surround the old main building. At noon, all of the churches in the area rang their bells to invoke a communal moment of silence for the hospital, followed by "Habeas Corpus," a sound installation for the entire main building of Northampton State Hospital. An extensive sound system was installed to animate the hollows of the architecture with J.S. Bach's *Magnificat,* as if they were the hollows of an instrument. Thousands of feet of cable were laid to connect all of the wings of the building. The loudspeakers were placed to sound with and through the space, as in this sunroom in the South Infirmary. (Above, courtesy of Hedwig Schüßler; below, courtesy of John Klondike Koehler.)

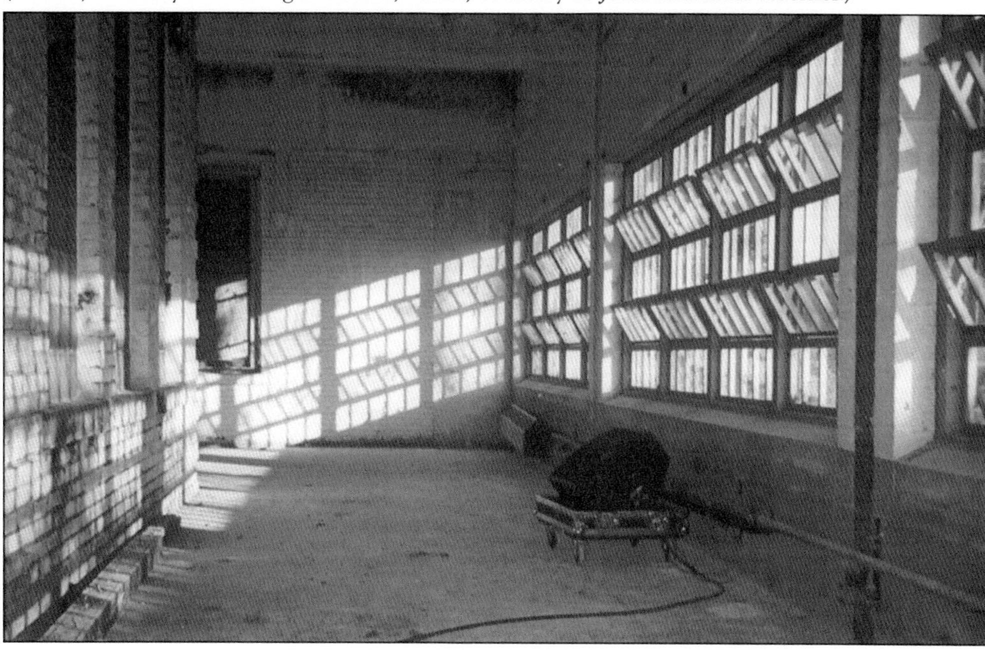

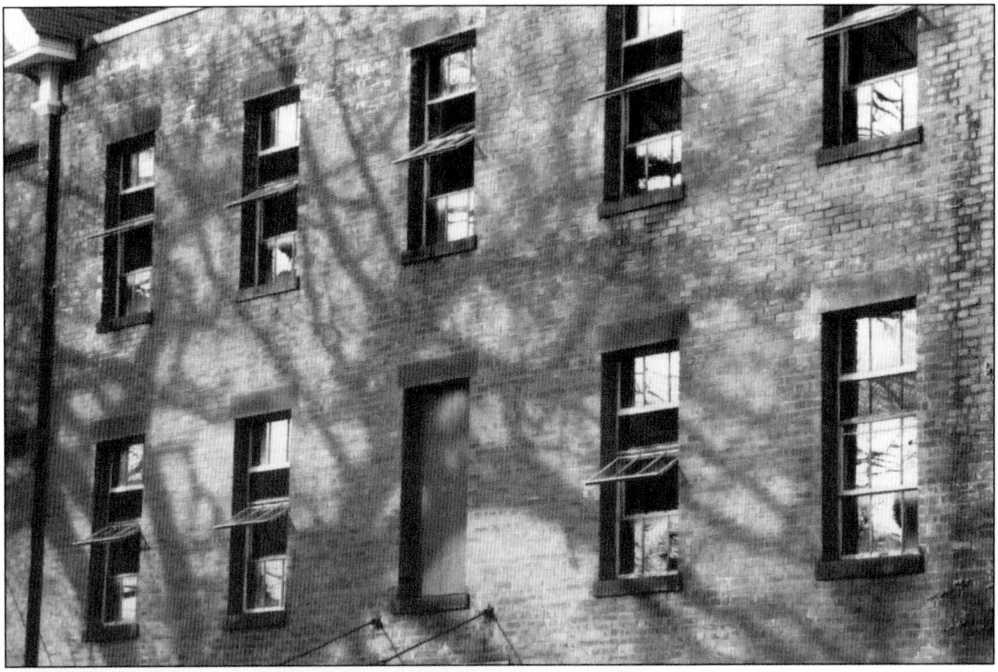

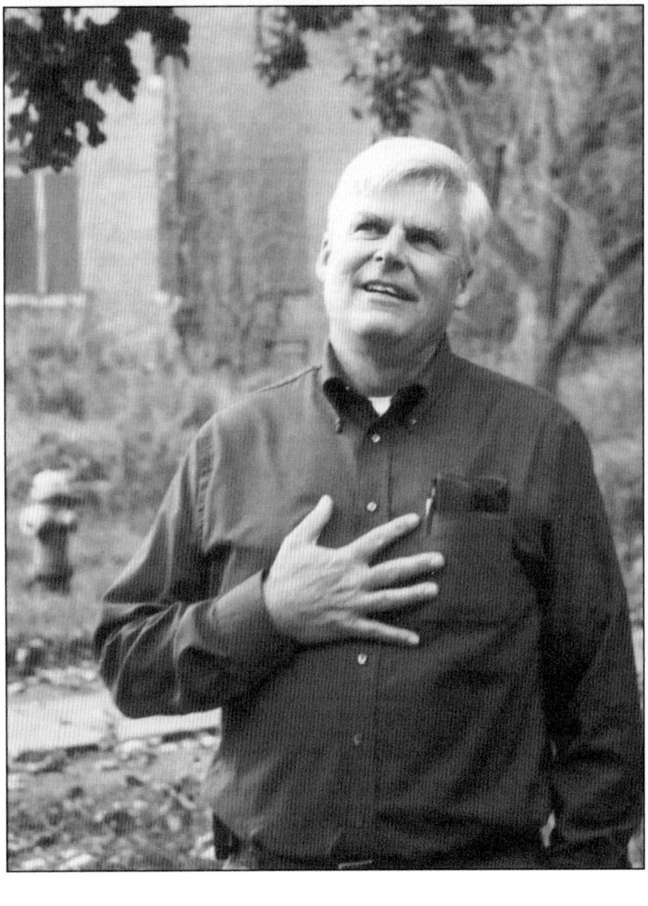

For the 28 minutes of the *Magnificat*, the building became a unified sound-body, reverberating and amplifying the choir and instruments of J.S. Bach, in a recording by Philippe Herreweghe/ Harmonia Mundi. Eighty volunteers helped to wire the building and open many hundreds of windows, which had not been opened in two decades. Longtime employee Kerry Holland was one of thousands who listened to the building sing. He was also part of the organizing committee of the events. (Both, courtesy of Hedwig Schüßler.)

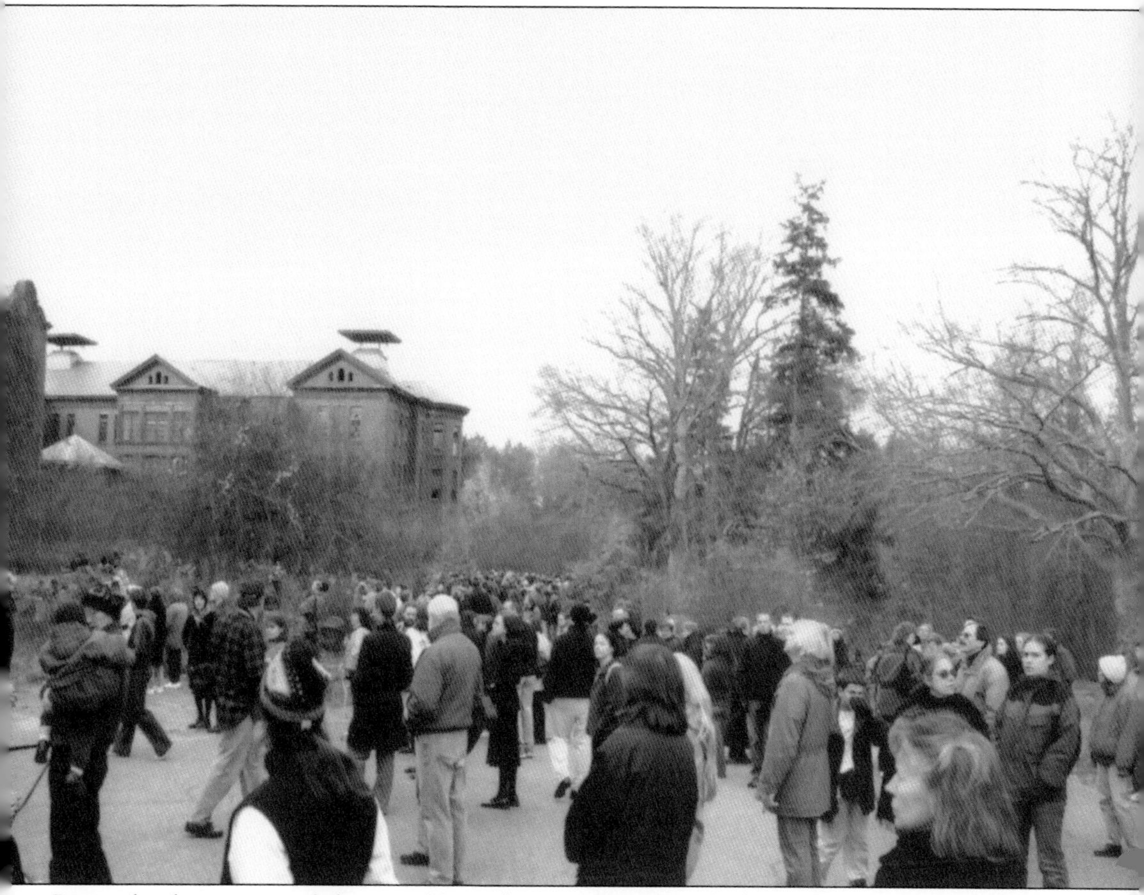

Pictured is the moment of silence on November 18, 2000, after which J.S. Bach's *Magnificat* began to ring through the architecture. Mayor Mary Clare Higgins declared a moment of silence with the following words: "Whereas, the Northampton State Hospital was founded in 1856 to receive persons who were suffering from mental illness; whereas, over the past one hundred and forty years, tens of thousands of persons suffered greatly at this institutions; whereas, the hospital has now been closed for almost a decade and we have embarked on a gentler and more individualized path of caring and supporting citizens with mental disabilities; now, therefore, I, the mayor of Northampton, hereby declare a moment of silence, to begin immediately following the ringing of church bells at midday on November 18, 2000, to remember the countless thousands of persons who suffered at the Northampton State Hospital, and the aspiration of our community to relieve that suffering in the most humane and caring way possible." (Courtesy of Hedwig Schüßler.)

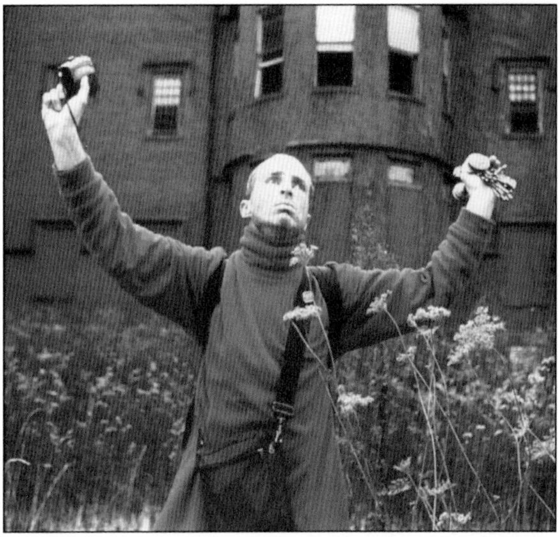

"If God allows it, I will be there for this unbelievable event," wrote Kermit S., a former patient, who had traveled up from Pennsylvania to be part of the events. He spoke at the patients' forum, and here, he is listening to the building during "Habeas Corpus." About the hospital, he said, "The idea supposedly was 'treatment.' However, when you speak of treatment you assume first of all there is something wrong with someone, and that there is something external that you can do to change that something. And then you assume that someone is therefore going to turn around and wind up living like everybody else on the outside again." (Courtesy of Paul Shoul.)

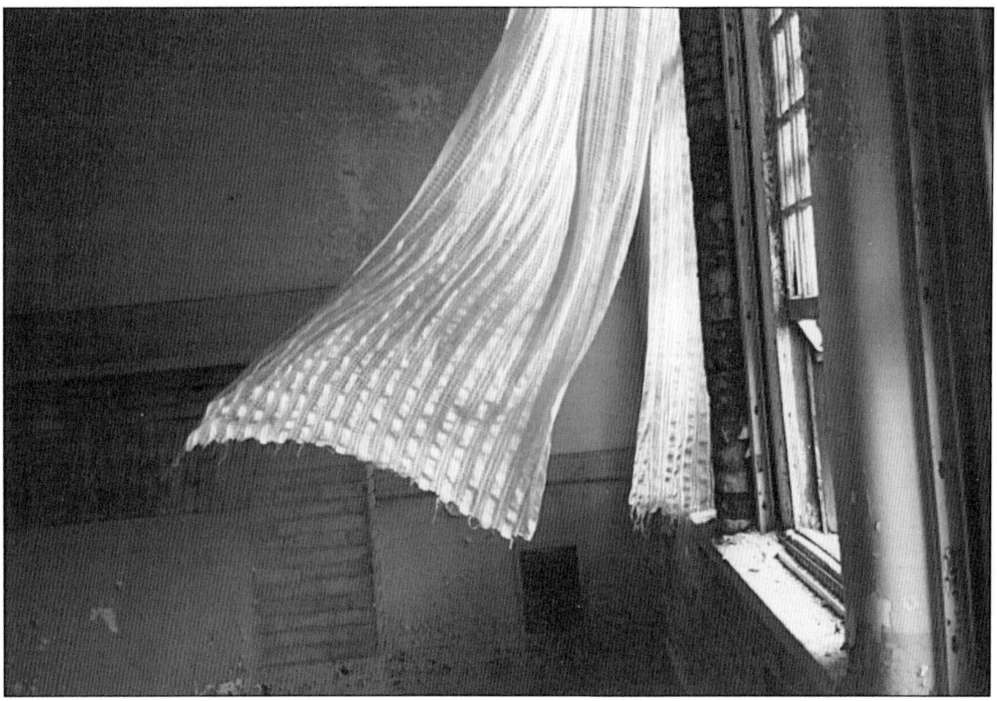

"I stood in the courtyard surrounded by South halls, and I thought of Lillian and Margo and Helen and Margaret, and all the other women I've worked with who spent decades of their lives at the hospital. White curtains fluttered in the open windows and the music spoke from inside those rooms. It felt as if, in that moment, their spirits were as whole and strong and fine as they might have been, and that the beauty and dignity that exists along with the tragedy and ruin of their lives was revealed," said Judy S., a volunteer during "Habeas Corpus," 2000. (Courtesy of Therese Schuleit.)

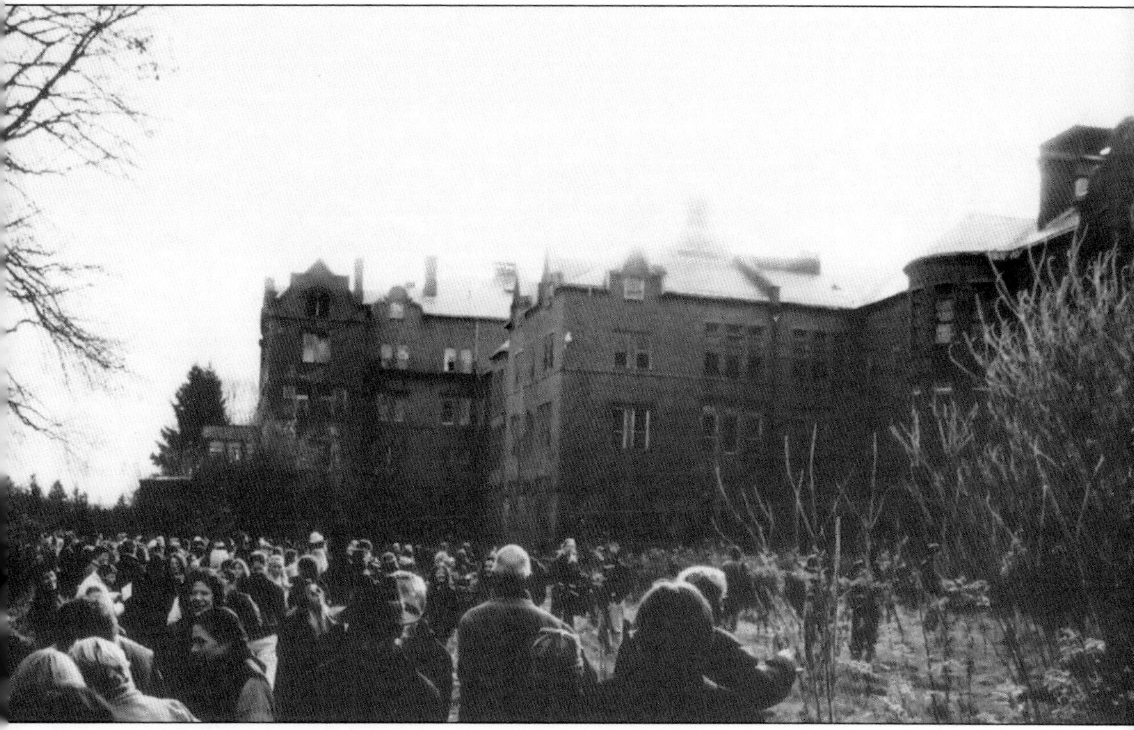

"The building exploded into glorious sound, as enveloping as headphones, and continued ringing for the full 28-minute duration. It echoed from the walls, it came from the sky, it seemed to emanate from everywhere and nowhere. An elderly, immaculately dressed woman stood off to one side and wept quietly throughout, tears cracking through her makeup. Meanwhile, a young man, as skilled and articulate as many a radio correspondent, read eager reports into his cassette recorder, describing 'Habeas Corpus' as the 'event of a lifetime.' And so it may have been. The faces in the crowd wore an infinity of expressions. This was a mass event that was also intimately personal; it seemed appropriate to greet your neighbor but not to watch too closely for any reactions. Far better to swim your own course through the sound and spirits," wrote Tim Page for the *Washington Post*. (Courtesy of Hedwig Schüßler.)

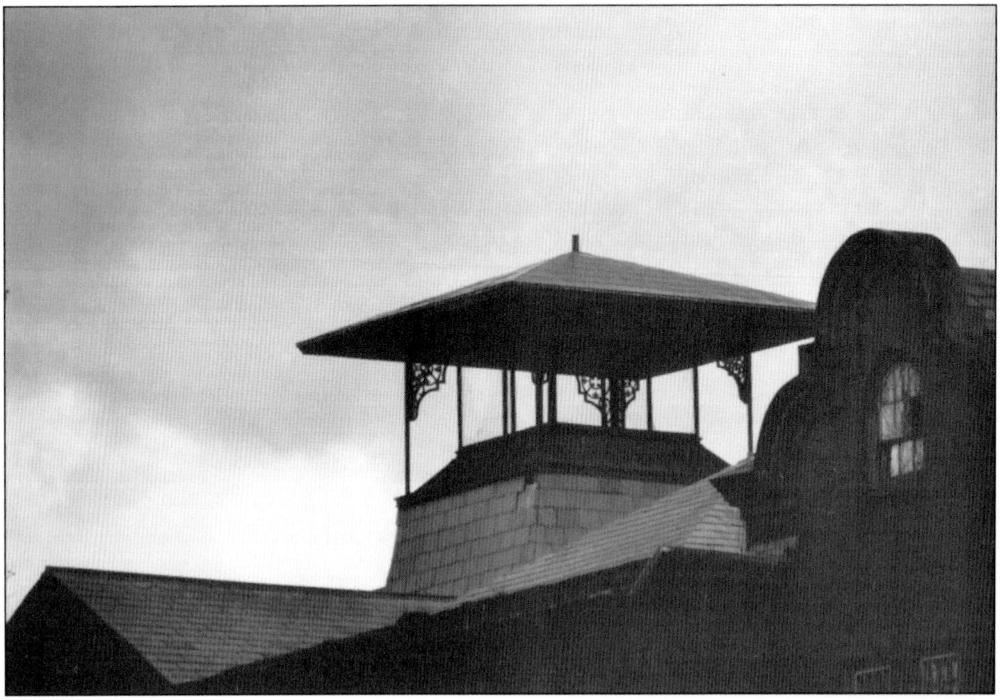

Many former patients and employees attended the memorial events in 2000. One employee had not seen the main building, which he knew so well, in over a decade. He said, "The condition of it is amazing, it's just terrible. There was a tremendous amount of torment here, and the building is also in torment right now. It looks like a sinking ship." (Both, courtesy of Therese Schuleit.)

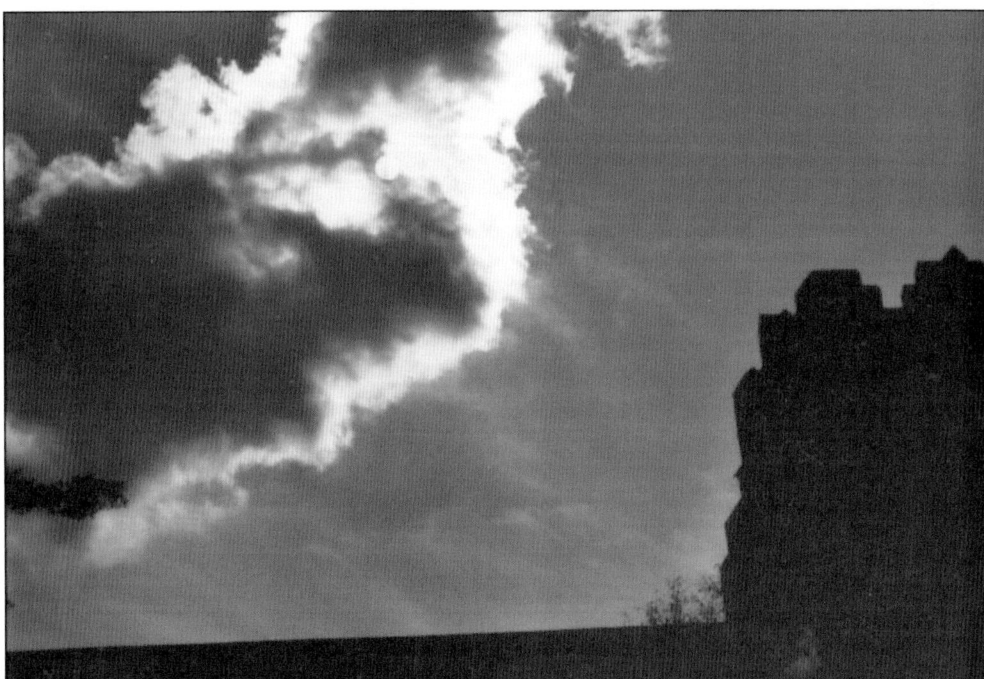

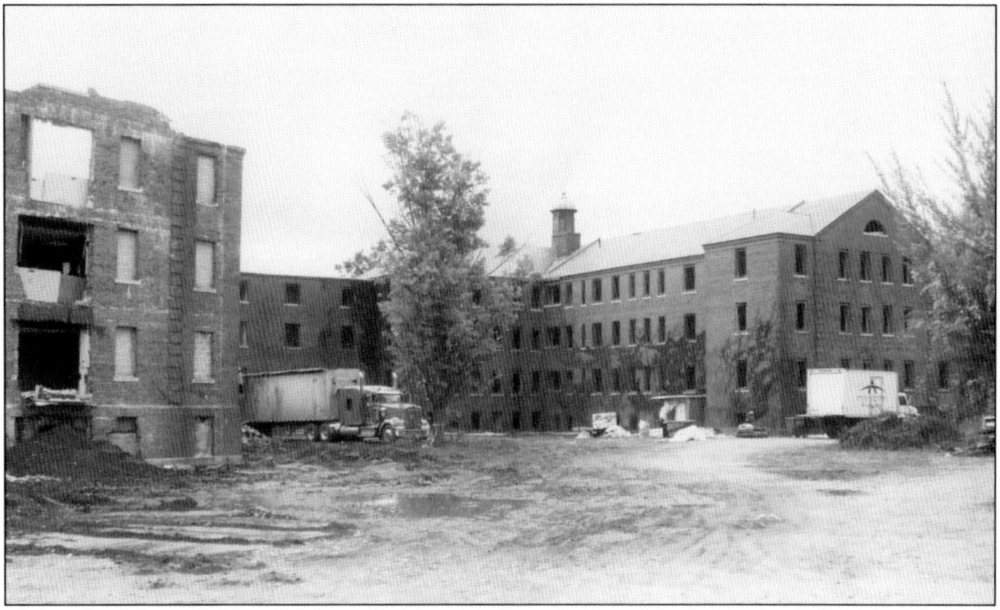

Demolition was under way in 2006. "My vision was that I would be there the day the big ball came and smacked the building and destroyed it. But the day that we moved my unit out of there, I cried my eyes out all day long. There was something very engaging and beautiful, and lovely, really, about that building. If we could have used it in the sort of tradition that it was built, we really would have had a beautiful hospital," reminisced a former employee.

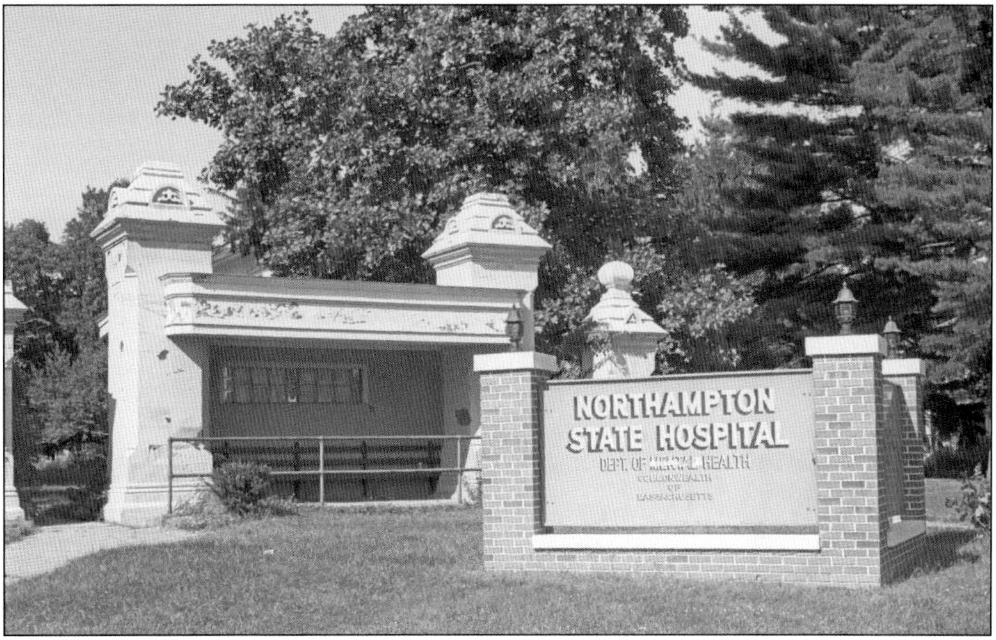

"We want to see that every car and truck that drives by will still know that this was the State Hospital. They could end up tearing down every single building that's up here. And then we will see absolutely nothing except this original entrance." As the hospital was closing, George Button Jr. spoke these words on behalf of workers pushing to create a memorial here. The 1867 entry gates had been transformed to a waiting area in 1945. (Courtesy of Stan Sherer.)

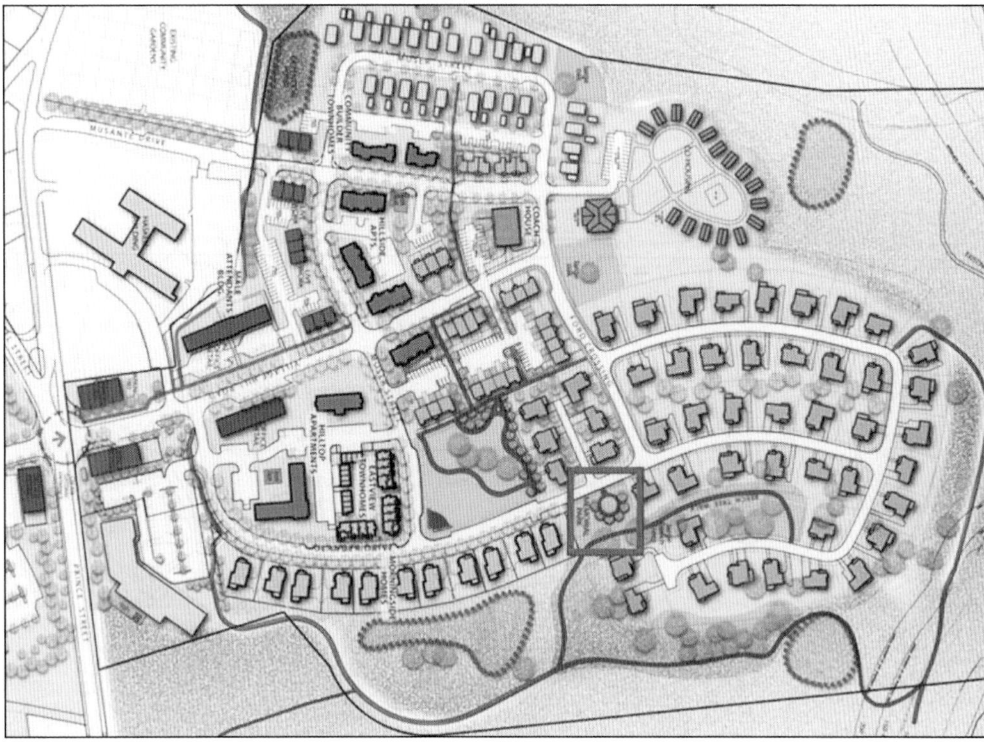

There was a long and sometimes contentious process to decide how the hospital and its grounds would be reused. MassDevelopment, a quasi-public agency, was chosen to lead the process. Early plans involved preserving the old main buildings, but time and money sealed their fate. Most of the historic structures have been demolished and replaced with new single-family housing, apartments, and industrial and commercial businesses. The South Home and the Nurses' Home were converted into the Hilltop Apartments in 2006. All of the original main hospital building has been torn down.

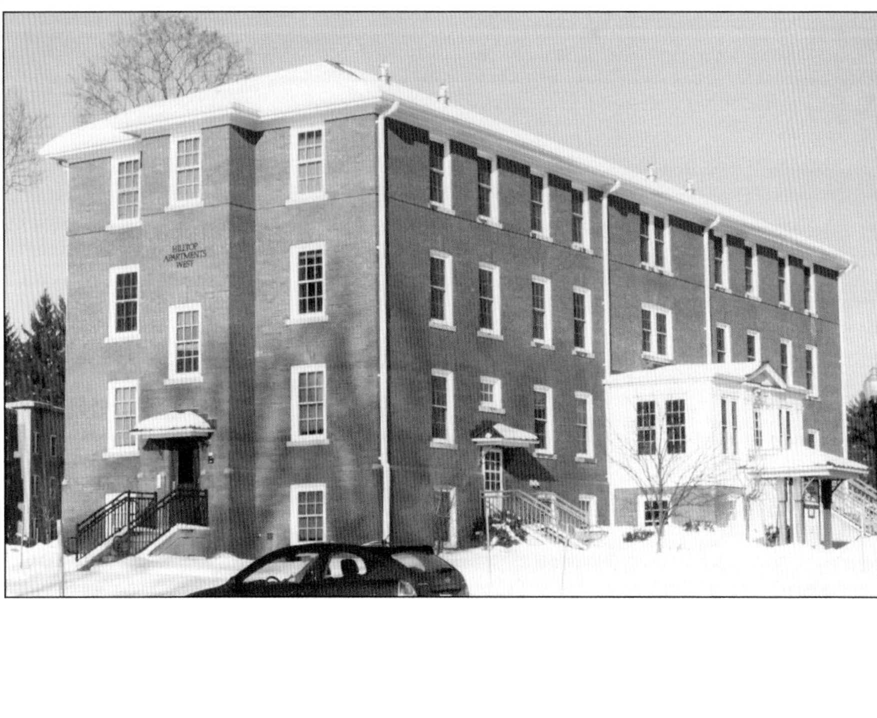

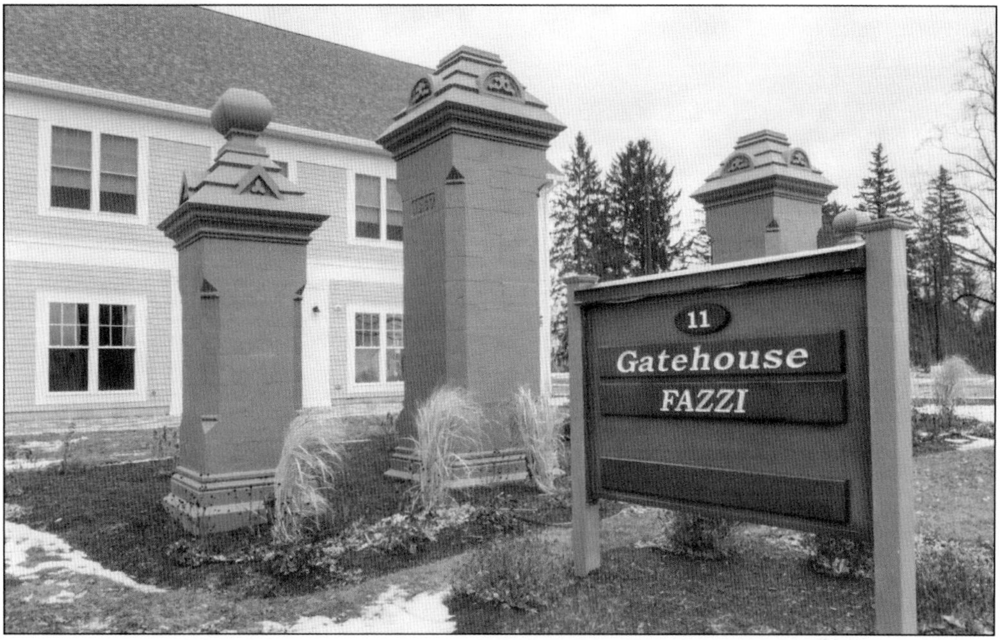

A new commercial office building, erected in 2013 behind the original gate, has taken its name. There is no indication of its historic role. The name of the redevelopment of the state hospital property has been changed from "Village on Hospital Hill" to "Village Hill of Northampton." (Courtesy of Stan Sherer.)

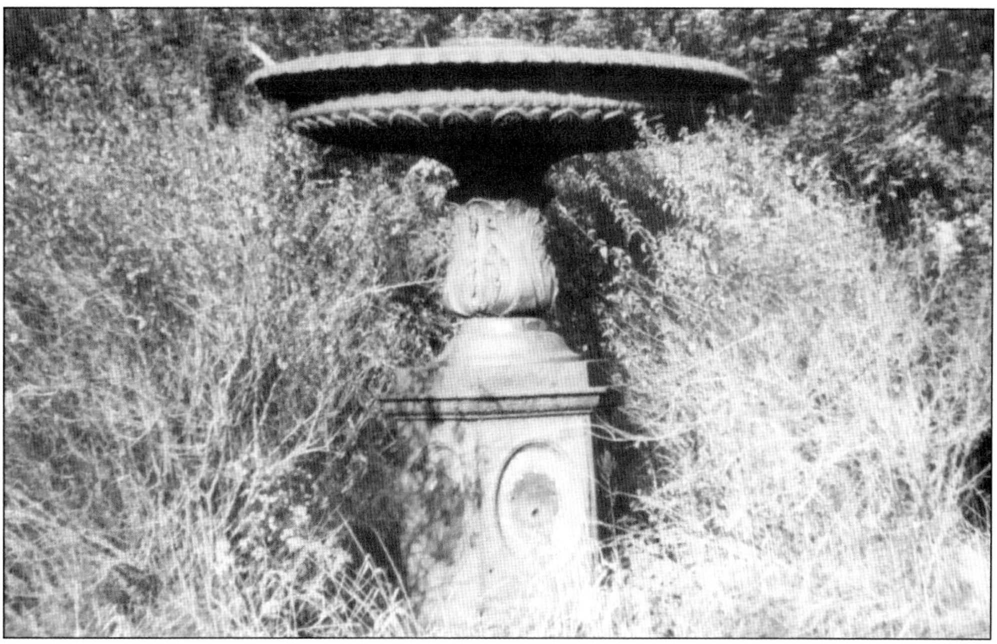
When the historic buildings were demolished to make way for new development, a group of concerned citizens formed to save the cast-iron fountain of the hospital. "This is the fountain of all the tears that have been shed at this hospital" was to be the inscription for the running fountain when reinstalled on its original site. Preservation efforts have gained steam with the award of a public grant to meet part of the cost.

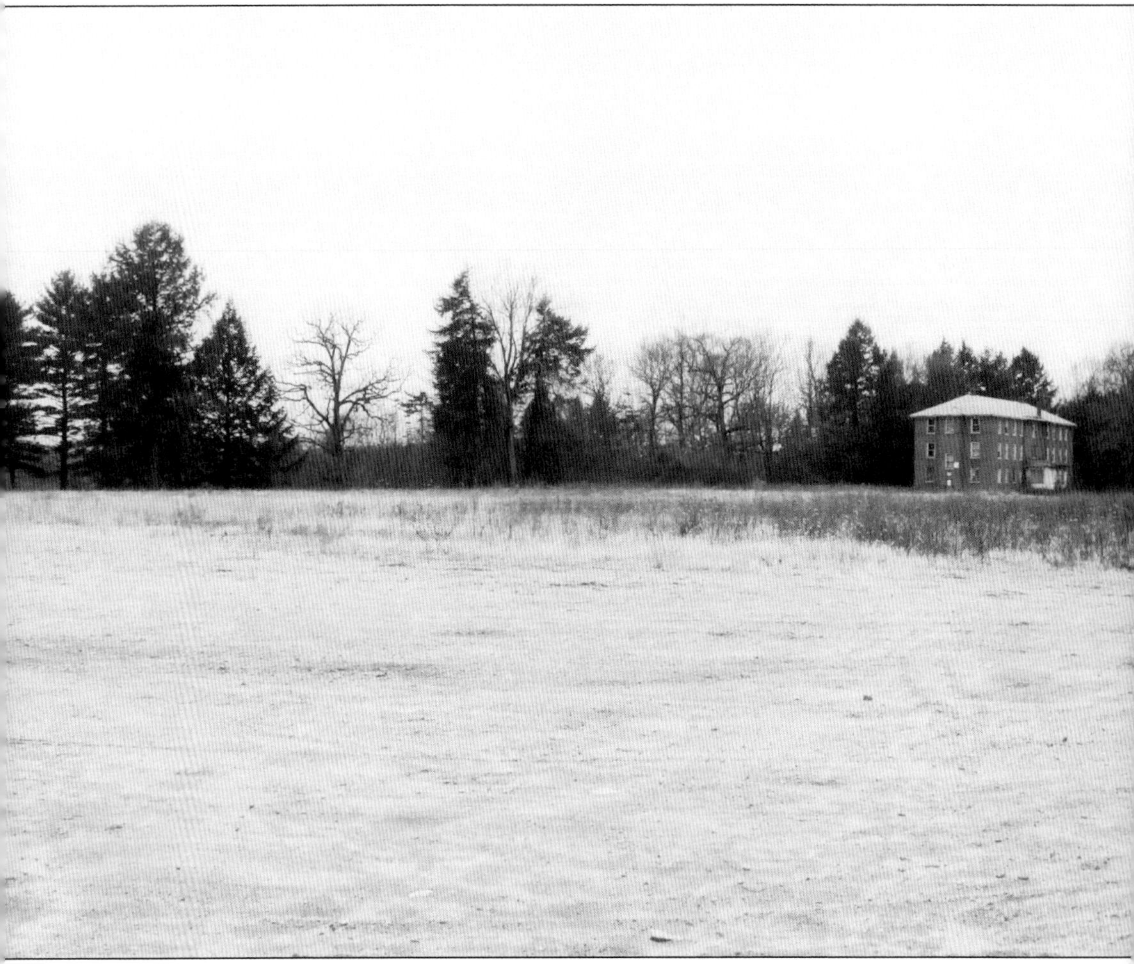

Despite being listed in the National Register of Historic Places, the buildings and grounds of Northampton State Hospital could not be saved. The main building had been without heat for 20 years and was too far gone—its demolition was inevitable. Also demolished, though visible in this 2008 picture, is the North Home, which served for decades as home to married employees. This is the site where the old main building once stood. A permanent physical memorial has not yet been created.

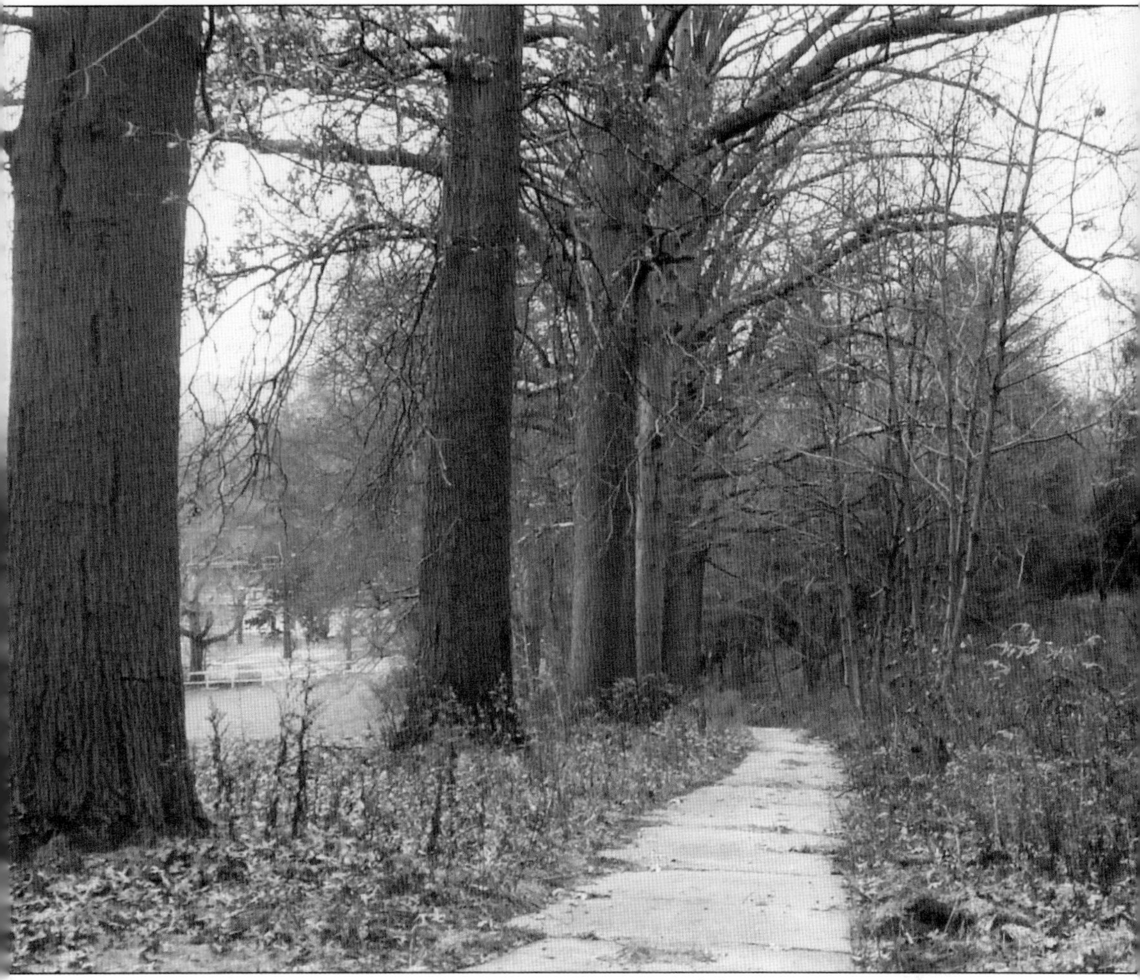

The old footpath that leads, to this day, from the hospital hill back into town is shown here. One employee remembers, "May we all be so blessed as to have the privilege to walk in someone else's shoes long enough to feel where they pinch. I will never forget E. who always tried to unlock the dayroom door by shaking it over and over. He incessantly swept the floor in between door-shaking episodes. Several years later I had the rare privilege of working as staff in the very community-based group home where E. was now living. And every evening E. would get up and unlock every door in the house. I understood in a deep way what he was doing: he was ensuring that he was free to come and go, no longer to be confined by a locked door that prevented his human right to the least restrictive environment possible. He was a blessing. He blessed me. It reminds me that no one can stop a person's spirit from the pursuit of happiness. The human soul cannot be confined, and no one could rob E. of his deepest human instinct to be free."